Praise for *A Smile to Change Your Life*

In my work with orthodontists all over the world, I have the pleasure of meeting exceptional clinicians and experts like Dr. James Crouse. In his book, A Smile to Change Your Life, *Dr. Crouse does a wonderful job explaining the benefits of orthodontic treatment for you or your child. This is a great resource to answer your questions straight from an orthodontic expert. I wish there was a book like this when I had braces years ago!*

— Dr. Dustin Burleson, Orthodontist and Founder of Burleson Seminars

Dr. Crouse's guidebook gives readers everything they need to know if they are considering orthodontic care for themselves or a loved one.

— Dr. John Burkett, DDS

A
SMILE
TO
CHANGE
YOUR LIFE

JAMES M. CROUSE, DDS

DIPLOMATE OF THE AMERICAN BOARD OF ORTHODONTICS

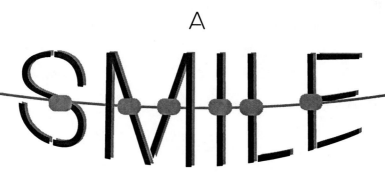

A SMILE TO CHANGE YOUR LIFE

A GUIDEBOOK TO ORTHODONTIC CARE

Advantage.

Published by Advantage, Charleston, South Carolina.
Member of Advantage Media Group.

ADVANTAGE is a registered trademark, and the Advantage colophon is a trademark of Advantage Media Group, Inc.

Printed in the United States of America.

10 9 8 7 6 5 4 3 2 1

ISBN: 978-1-59932-850-8
LCCN: 2017942416

Cover design by Katie Biondo.
Layout design by Megan Elger.

This publication is designed to provide accurate and authoritative information in regard to the subject matter covered. It is sold with the understanding that the publisher is not engaged in rendering legal, accounting, or other professional services. If legal advice or other expert assistance is required, the services of a competent professional person should be sought.

Advantage Media Group is proud to be a part of the Tree Neutral® program. Tree Neutral offsets the number of trees consumed in the production and printing of this book by taking proactive steps such as planting trees in direct proportion to the number of trees used to print books. To learn more about Tree Neutral, please visit **www.treeneutral.com.**

Advantage Media Group is a publisher of business, self-improvement, and professional development books. We help entrepreneurs, business leaders, and professionals share their Stories, Passion, and Knowledge to help others Learn & Grow. Do you have a manuscript or book idea that you would like us to consider for publishing? Please visit **advantagefamily.com** or call **1.866.775.1696.**

To Susan, my wife, business partner, and best friend.

Table of Contents

ACKNOWLEDGMENTS

I want to thank the people who helped make this book possible—the patients and their families who have graced my office and entrusted me to treat their most precious possessions. My effort to educate these people is the main impetus for writing this book. I'd also like to thank people like Dan Kennedy, Dustin Burleson, Adam Witty, and the other excellent people at Advantage Media who helped me believe that this was something I could accomplish. Finally, many thanks to my team for supporting me with stories and ideas that helped give the book life.

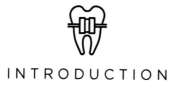

MORE THAN JUST A NICE SMILE

If I've learned one undeniable pearl of wisdom during my more than twenty-five years as a practicing orthodontist, it's that honest, transparent dialogue between a doctor and his patient is a critical first step in achieving successful outcomes. The more straightforward I can be—the more clearly I can communicate what I'm doing and why I'm doing it to my patients—the greater the chance for truly favorable results.

I know that most of my patients come to my office with a set of preconceived notions as to what will happen during their visit. And I realize that some of my patients are genuinely fearful of what may lie ahead.

That's only human—and completely understandable. We all fear the unknown.

Think, for example, of when you've been on an airplane, sitting on the tarmac, assuming that your flight will take off at its designated time, only to realize it's not going to leave as scheduled. It's an unsettling feeling, isn't it? No one knows what's going on or what exactly is causing the delay, so people just sit there brooding in the dark. Some get nervous, others irritated. Their imaginations get the better of them, until someone has the courtesy to announce what is happening and—more importantly—*why* it's happening. When questions are answered and people stay informed, they bring down their defenses, allowing proper adjustments to be made.

I sincerely believe that you, as a patient, deserve the very same level of communication when you have your teeth examined.

When it comes to orthodontic work, I don't believe in keeping people in the dark, stranded on some metaphorical runway. I *want* people to ask me questions. And I believe in the importance of answering them with as much clarity as possible.

By this time, I know which questions tend to arise more often than others. Will the procedure hurt? How long will it take? What are you going to do? How long do I have to keep my mouth open?

And if you're a parent or adult, the dreaded questions: *Does my child need braces? How much will this cost? And how am I going to pay for it?*

The truth of the matter is that I wrote *A Smile to Change Your Life* because I've long wanted to give my patients a succinct, easily digestible guidebook on orthodontic care, but could never find one I was satisfied with. I consider this book to be a reference tool for anyone who is considering orthodontic treatments. Teens. Adults. Seniors. Parents. Anyone.

I've attempted to write in a style that mirrors the kind of conversations that my patients and I share in my office. It has been written to try to replace common myths surrounding orthodontic treatment with practical knowledge and trusted advice.

Ultimately, I hope that what is contained within these pages will make you a better consumer and help you to avoid many of the pitfalls I've seen people face over the years. If any part of this book helps you make the right decisions for you and your family, then I will have achieved my primary goal.

Let me begin, therefore, by addressing some of the questions you might have about this book in general.

WHY SHOULD I READ THIS BOOK?

Receiving proper orthodontic treatments can quite literally change your life. I say this from personal experience, having seen so many of my patients rise out of my chair with a beautiful new smile and a newfound sense of confidence. And while there are aesthetic advantages to orthodontic work, there are also health benefits that most people are simply unaware of. The health of one's teeth, jaw, and mouth can contribute not only to common problems like cavities and gum disease, but also to more serious issues, like heart attacks and strokes in adults, as well as ADHD and bed-wetting in children.

The truth is that orthodontic treatment is a major investment, so you have to be on guard against wasting your money. There are several different options available to you in terms of orthodontic care. The key, in my mind, is for you to be an informed consumer and be able to discern quality information from the disinformation that is out there.

How, for instance, do you know if your doctor is a good one? Your orthodontics provider could be a well-respected member of the dental community with years of training and experience, or someone who just returned from a weekend course on the subject. Please keep in mind that very little

Please keep in mind that very little orthodontics is taught in dental school, which brings us to our first myth.

orthodontics is taught in dental school, which brings us to our first myth.

MYTH 1: ALL ORTHODONTIC TREATMENT IS THE SAME.

Let me begin by sharing a personal anecdote. One day, a nice young woman with a set of noticeably crooked front teeth found her way to my office. Happy days were ahead for her. She was getting married and wanted to ensure she had a nice smile for her wedding photos.

She had wanted to straighten her teeth for some time. In fact, years earlier, she had told her dentist about her wishes, and he had responded by telling her that she didn't even need to leave his chair. He promised her he could improve her smile by using clear aligners in just a few months. She was both relieved and excited, and she happily agreed to begin treatment. Why not? She didn't have to go to another office with some doctor she didn't know. She could be treated in familiar, comfortable surroundings.

Flash forward two years and countless impressions and trays later, and her teeth and smile remained virtually unchanged. When she came to my office and told me her story, we talked about her history, and I discovered that her dentist had used a less-expensive aligner system. That was mistake number one. More egregious was the fact that he had attempted to treat a problem that is especially difficult to correct with aligners. It can be done, but it takes an expert. He was attempting to treat a problem that the majority of ortho-dontists would not attempt with aligners. He simply didn't have the knowledge to realize he was in over his head.

I met her in January, with her wedding set for that very summer. "Can you fix me in time for my wedding?" she asked, nervously. I told her it wouldn't be easy—especially considering the limited amount of time we had to work with—but that I knew the best approach to pursue.

Fortunately, with the help of accelerated orthodontic treatment, we were able to get her front teeth aligned so that she had a gorgeous smile for her wedding photos. And she lived, as the fairy tales tell us, happily ever after.

We dentists tend to be perfectionists. We are accustomed to success most of the time, so it can be hard for some of us to admit defeat and ask for help from specialists. But that's exactly what needed to be done in the case of this patient.

The big picture takeaway lesson of my story is that dentists and orthodontists are two entirely different health care professionals. Orthodontics is the first dental specialty and the second health care specialty (ophthalmology was the first), very different from all other aspects of dentistry. An orthodontist is a dentist who has gone back to school, in a university setting, for an additional two to three years of study. We have taken classes specifically focused on growth and development, malocclusion (crooked teeth, bad bite), and the proper techniques for straightening teeth. That's all that we, as orthodontists, do. We don't handle fillings or crowns or clean teeth, so patients still need a general dentist to take care of their overall dental health. Together, your general dentist and the orthodontist partner to ensure that you receive the best care possible.

MYTH 2: ORTHODONTIC TREATMENT IS ONLY FOR TEENAGERS.

Nothing could be further from the truth. The American Association of Orthodontists, for instance, recommends that children be evaluated for the first time at age seven, a time when most children's four upper and four lower incisors have come in, as well as the time when first permanent molars have also come in.

At that age, what we're really looking at is whether those teeth are actually there. We're looking at the position of the developing teeth, checking for missing teeth or even extra teeth. Should a child's jaw be too narrow, it can contribute to breathing problems. I am looking for any conditions that, if left untreated, will cause damage or make future treatment more complicated. Early treatment can prevent the need for removal of permanent teeth and even avoid the need for jaw surgery! Whatever the case, it's beneficial for children to be seen by an orthodontist before all of their baby teeth fall out, as we are experts in the growth and development of teeth and the jaws. There are still dentists and hygienists who believe that all the baby teeth need to be gone before referring a child to the orthodontist. This is a big mistake and often severely limits the treatment options available.

If I don't identify a problem that requires immediate attention, then I put patients in our monitoring system. We see them periodically. We monitor their growth, making sure their baby teeth are falling out on time. If an extraction is required, it's better to handle it earlier rather than later, as proper early interventions will allow permanent teeth to develop in the proper place at the proper time. If treatment is indicated, it can be done at the right time so that treatment is quick and efficient (and less expensive).

I have treated children as young as four years old to correct cross bites that forced them to bite abnormally. Fortunately, early treatments are usually relatively quick and simple. Correction of a cross bite can be accomplished in as little as one month. This simple correction can make a world of difference in the future.

One word of caution: *Early treatment will NOT ensure that a child won't need full braces when the permanent teeth come in.* As I stated earlier, it's to prevent damage and make future treatment easier.

MYTH 3: ORTHODONTIC TREATMENT IS ONLY FOR IMPROVING A PERSON'S SMILE.

As important as a nice smile may be, many people are under the incorrect assumption that orthodontic treatments are performed strictly to make people look more attractive, like plastic surgery for people who feel their noses are too big or their cheeks need tightening.

While it's true that orthodontic treatment does result in a fuller, more beautiful smile, orthodontists are also responsible for ensuring that teeth fit together so that they function optimally. When the teeth fit together well, what we call a proper bite, they are able to chew effectively. Straight teeth, for example, are less susceptible to adverse tooth wear, reduce the risk of temporomandibular joint (TMJ) problems, and help patients chew efficiently and breathe more easily. Crooked teeth and uneven bites, by contrast, put people more at risk for gum (periodontal) disease, extensive restorative work (fillings, crowns), and even root canals.

Should a tooth need to be restored, a dentist can do a much better job if the teeth are in the correct alignment. Sometimes the way a person's teeth fit together causes him or her to have to shift the jaw to one side or another. This can cause adverse forces on the teeth and puts strain on the jaw muscles and jaw joints. If you combine this with stress, then you have a recipe for disease. Straight teeth and a good bite are an important part of overall good oral health.

WHAT IS INVISALIGN?

At some point, you might have heard of an increasingly popular product called Invisalign, without quite knowing exactly what it is. Here's the most basic definition I can provide: Invisalign is a removable appliance (like a mouth guard) that is used for orthodontic treatment as opposed to traditional braces, which are attached to the teeth and cannot be removed by the patient.

Invisalign has slowly gained acceptance by orthodontists in the United States. However, most orthodontists only treat 20 percent of their patients with Invisalign versus 80 percent with traditional braces. Orthodontists, like most people, want to stay in their comfort zone—and their comfort zone is traditional braces. They are willing to treat simple cases with Invisalign, but for anything beyond that, they like to stick with what they know. Often, they will tell people that they are not candidates for Invisalign and steer them into traditional braces. There are orthodontists who have embraced (no pun intended) this new technology and have stretched the limits. In my office, I am as comfortable treating all orthodontic problems with Invisalign as I am treating them with traditional braces. I'm proud to say that I'm in the top 1 percent of Invisalign providers in North America.

The aligners are very thin, like bleaching trays, and are custom-made for your teeth. The process involves using a series of trays that slowly move your teeth. The trays are changed weekly on your own, and patients are typically given enough trays to last six to eight weeks. The visits to the orthodontist are quick and easy. The fit of the aligners is checked, and you are given more aligners.

In my opinion, there are many advantages to using Invisalign. The aligners are practically invisible, there is little or no discomfort, there are no eating restrictions, and it is very easy for patients to clean their teeth. It's the wave of the future.

MYTH 4: ORTHODONTIC WORK IS PROHIBITIVELY EXPENSIVE.

I'm often asked the question, "How much do braces cost?" And although I understand the desire for a simple answer, the truth of the matter is that the expense of orthodontic work varies based on a patient's particular needs.

Asking orthodontists how much their services will cost is a little like asking a boat dealer how much a boat costs. The honest answer is that it depends. A boat dealer needs to know what kind of vessel you actually want—an inflatable raft or a luxury yacht.

In a similar fashion, orthodontists can only begin to estimate how much appropriate treatments will cost after you come in for an examination. Fortunately, most orthodontists offer inexpensive or complimentary orthodontic exams. All you need to do is make an appointment.

You should know that the fee for braces is often based on a number of variables. There is often, for example, a fee for the creation of orthodontic records as well as the actual cost of the treatment. Some orthodontists charge a separate fee for removing braces and retainers. This is important because if you are doing comparison shopping, you need to know what is included in the fee that you are presented. I encourage my patients to thoroughly vet those estimates. Is there, for instance, a charge for missed appointments, broken brackets, or treatments that are taking longer than expected? Are there different retainer options? If you are comparing the prices of treatments, make sure you are comparing oranges to oranges and not oranges to apples.

One other very important thing to remember: You typically don't pay by the number of times you visit someone's office. The fee you are quoted should be for the entire service. Payment over the course of the treatment, in terms of financing, is done as a convenience to make treatments more affordable. In our office, we offer a full range of different pre-payment discounts and financings options.

Most orthodontists break the cost of orthodontic treatment into an initial payment and then monthly payments over the course of the treatment. There is no interest charged. Some people don't have the ready cash for a sizable down payment. There are outside finance companies that will loan others the money for orthodontic treatment so that patients can just make a monthly payment. Many of these are interest-free for up to two years.

You typically don't pay by the number of times you visit someone's office. The fee you are quoted should be for the entire service.

Whatever payment system you agree to, just remember that you must make your payments every month as agreed upon, whether you are seen that month or not. You pay your car payment every month whether you drive it all day or let it sit in a garage. The same expectations exist in the orthodontic world.

WHAT I HOPE YOU TAKE FROM THIS BOOK

My central hope is that by reading this book you will be a better consumer: more knowledgeable, more empowered, and better equipped to make decisions that you feel comfortable about. I want your experience to be positive and make you feel like it was the best money you've ever spent.

When I was a boy, I absolutely hated going to the dentist's office. While in my dentist's office, I quickly learned how to distinguish between a "drill" and a "tooth cleaner." No one told me what was coming, so if I saw a tooth cleaner sitting on my dentist's instrument table, I was fine. But when I saw a drill sitting there, I got worried. I keep this in mind when my patients are sitting in the chair. I don't want them sitting there worried about what is going to happen to them.

But I have equally vivid memories of my trips to the orthodontist, which were a completely different experience altogether. At the time, I tended to associate the dental office with elevator music. But when I went to my orthodontist, I found that he was playing the same radio station that my friends and I listened to. He had issues of *MAD Magazine* in the waiting room as well as caring, attractive women as assistants—an undeniable plus for a teenage boy.

I actually looked forward to my orthodontic appointments. For me, there was no stigma attached to wearing braces. It seemed like everyone in school had them, and I wanted to be like my friends. I never felt pain when I was sitting in my orthodontist's office. And while my teeth did get a little sore after adjustments, there was never any dread involved. I even got out of school every month to have my braces adjusted. After two years, I could physically see what his treatments had done. My teeth were straight! This changed my perception of myself as well as of dentistry in general.

I hope after paging through *A Smile to Change Your Life*—and undergoing quality orthodontic treatment—that your own perspectives will change in a similar fashion.

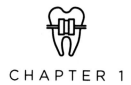

HOW DO I FIND THE BEST ORTHODONTIST?

Hello, Dear Reader! Chapter 1 explores:

- *Choosing an Orthodontic Plan*
- *My Golden Rules for Treating a Patient*
- *Where Do I Begin When Searching for an Orthodontist?*
- *How Should I Prepare for My First Visit?*
- *A Virtual Tour of Our Office*
- *What Should I Look for In an Initial Evaluation*
- *Top-Ten Questions to Ask Your Orthodontist*
- *Payment Options and Flexible Financing*
- *Getting a Second Opinion*

Preparing for orthodontic treatment is a lot like planning a long road trip in a foreign country. You will inevitably make the most important decisions before your journey even begins.

While abroad, you will need to hire someone who has a real sense for the lay of the land—someone who knows both the thoroughfares and back roads that are going to get you where you need to go as safely, efficiently, and painlessly as possible. Do you want to hire an amateur valet—some former Uber driver who wants to branch out into bigger and better assignments—or someone who knows the various routes to your destination like the back of his hand?

You also want someone who can provide you options along the way, someone who knows more than one possible route toward your given destination and understands what to do when mechanical problems arise or road closures emerge, so that you don't run into any unforeseen issues. You'll have to ask him the vital question: Can you seamlessly change paths at a moment's notice?

You need to do research. Will your driver of choice be reliable? How many times—and with how many people—has he made the journey? What does the vehicle look like? Is it up-to-date in terms of the latest technologies and creature comforts that are going to make your journey as enjoyable as possible?

And you'll want to ensure that he will be able to drive you precisely where you want to go. Getting to Quebec is one thing. Getting to that lovely, hard-to-find B&B on the road to Montreal is something else entirely. In other words, you don't want a driver who will turn to you at some point and say, "Unfortunately, this is as far as I can get you."

Not to mention the fact that you want to find someone who you will enjoy sharing the journey with: someone you can talk to—and who will talk with you, guide you to the right spots, and maybe even educate you along the way.

When it comes to choosing an orthodontist, whether it's me or some other highly skilled practitioner, it's imperative that you pursue a similar strategy. Ask questions. And see how potential candidates respond. Any orthodontist who struggles to answer your initial questions in a satisfactory way is almost certain to leave you feeling cold and uninformed later in your treatment.

You want to go to an orthodontist who has chosen to make the investments necessary to obtain and use the latest technologies, primarily because it is those very technologies that will make your experience—as a patient—more convenient, comfortable, and efficient.

I've embarked on many journeys with my patients over the years and hope that the following chapter will give you a clear road map of how effective orthodontists approach the initial stages of their consultations with patients.

CHOOSING AN ORTHODONTIC TREATMENT PLAN

Let's look at an example. Your twelve-year-old son has crooked teeth and an overbite. There are three orthodontists in town. You are a smart consumer so you decide you will shop around and find the doc that will give you the best price.

The first doctor has been in practice for fifty years. The office is decorated like it's been stuck in a time warp and never evolved past 1972. He has spit sinks with rust stains. He does an exam on Junior and says he needs braces for two years, four bicuspids removed, and he needs to wear a headgear (night brace) ten to fourteen hours per day. Your son asks about treatment with Invisalign and is told he is absolutely *not* a candidate.

The next orthodontist has been out of training for a year. She looks at Junior and says that he needs braces, but he doesn't need any teeth removed. She says she will correct his overbite with a Herbst appliance that is entirely inside the mouth and that there is nothing that he has to put on or remove. He also needs an expander.

Treatment time will be approximately two years. She also says that he is not a candidate for Invisalign.

At the third orthodontist, you are given the option of traditional braces or Invisalign and the removal of two upper bicuspids.

The costs of the various treatments are similar, perhaps within a few hundred dollars.

Your head is spinning: You have seen three doctors and been given three very different treatment plans. Which one is right and which one is wrong? That is one of the truisms about orthodontic treatments. There are a number of different ways to get from point A to point B, and it's not merely that one is right and the other is wrong. In the end, you simply have to feel comfortable about both the plan and the doctor.

Let's look at another example. This time, you are the one wanting to straighten your teeth.

The first orthodontist takes a look and tells you that you indeed would benefit from orthodontic treatment. You have crowding and an "overbite." You require full traditional braces and will need to have two permanent teeth removed.

The second one agrees with the first doctor but tells you that instead of having teeth removed, you need to have jaw surgery to move your lower jaw out. "What? Jaw surgery?" you say. "I just want my teeth straightened."

The third orthodontist says that, yes, you have an "overbite," but if that doesn't bother you, then we can treat you without removing teeth or doing surgery.

Which one is right? This is where having clear goals is important. We doctors have an obligation to offer the ideal treatment, and there are many of my colleagues who only want to perform what they consider to be an "ideal" treatment. Compromised treatment is where the result is not perfect from the orthodontist's standpoint, but it's an improvement, and that improvement may be the only thing that was bothering the patient in the first place. The important thing, from my perspective, is for you to know your options and what results you want to get out of going through orthodontic treatment.

MY GOLDEN RULES FOR TREATING A PATIENT

Good communication is critical for a good result and positive experience. The doctor has an obligation to inform you of your condition, the treatment options, and how your treatment is progressing. It's also important for the patient to be comfortable asking the doctor any questions regarding the treatment. This kind of two-way communication ensures that there are no surprises.

Doctors in the past were authority figures who dispensed orders that were to be obeyed and never questioned. They were not easy people to have conversations with. Fortunately, that paternalistic style is disappearing. Health care is more and more a collaborative effort between the doctor and the patient.

I make a sincere effort to keep lines of communication open between myself, my patients, and the parents.

Probably the most common question going through a patient's mind is "When am I getting my braces off?" There has been more than one occasion where I've caused tears by telling a young lady that her braces aren't coming off today—even though to her, the teeth look straight. Although she might have come a long way from the crooked teeth that sent her to my office in the first place, I am able to explain—and show—where she will be when the procedures are finished.

The typical orthodontic office can be described as controlled chaos. There is an open bay with several chairs full of patients with the doctor running from one chair to another. This allows us to treat a lot of patients and keep our costs down and your treatment affordable. The downside is that it can feel dehumanizing—as though you're being run through an assembly line. However, we make it a point to remember that there are *people* attached to the teeth we are working on—patients who are often wondering what the heck is going on but don't want to be a bother. Therefore, it's a priority in my office to keep the patient and parent informed about what we are doing, how the treatment is progressing, and what the plan is for the next appointment. It's also why we welcome parents into the treatment area so they know what is going on with their children.

WHERE DO I BEGIN WHEN SEARCHING FOR AN ORTHODONTIST?

I encourage you, whether you plan on visiting my office or not, to investigate whether your doctor of choice is a member of the American Association of Orthodontists. Only orthodontists can be members of this organization. The providers of weekend courses on orthodontics give out certificates that make it *look* like dentists have had sufficient training in orthodontics. Often, though, they simply have not.

> *Investigate whether your doctor of choice is a member of the American Association of Orthodontists.*

Once you have decided to see an orthodontist, remember to ask questions.

Personally, I am extraordinarily invested in making sure that we—as doctor and patient—select the best treatment options for you. I consider it my job to tell you what I think the best treatment will be and what it will take to get you there. These treatment plans may involve years of braces and jaw surgery. But chances are, you're less concerned about my interpretation of what a perfect result might be and more concerned about what *your* vision for a successful treatment is. I promise you that no matter the circumstances, I will try to honor your definition as to what constitutes a "successful treatment."

You may, for instance, want straight teeth, and the fact that you have a little bit of an "overbite" does not bother you in the least. That's fine. For some, an attractive smile is the sole goal. For others, aesthetic considerations will take a back seat to exploring how we can relieve pain or help treat particular health issues. At the end of the day, I believe it's my responsibility to inform and educate you—then step back and let you decide what treatment is best for *you*.

At my office, we don't believe in or ascribe to high-pressure tactics. Never have and never will.

HOW SHOULD I PREPARE FOR MY FIRST VISIT?

Your initial examination with an orthodontist will vary from doctor to doctor, but at our office we have a set procedure that we've developed over the twenty-five-plus years I've been in practice.

We try to be as proactive as we can with paperwork. When you make an appointment at my office, we send you documents to complete prior to your visit. This includes a medical history, insurance information, and some information about my practice and the office. The forms can be filled out online as well.

We do this because I don't believe in the modern "clipboard" approach to medicine, handing you a bunch of forms to fill out in a crowded waiting room. We do our best to come to you, welcome you by name, and help you get comfortable.

When you arrive for your appointment, you will be warmly greeted by one of our team members and then given a tour of the office. This is our way of helping you to get to know us a little better and lets us show off our office, which we are quite proud of.

A VIRTUAL TOUR OF OUR OFFICE

Our office has been designed to be bright, cheerful, and fun. I love it when people say they've never been in a doctor's office that looks like ours. It's a modern space, complete with the latest technologies, which means your treatment will be completed as efficiently—and with the least amount of disruption to your daily routine—as possible. We take into consideration your schedule, where you live, and if there are other family members in treatment, so you aren't making any more trips to our office than is necessary.

Unlike some doctors, I always encourage parents to come into the back to our treatment area with their children so that they know what we are doing, how treatments are progressing, and what they need to be doing, including brushing better or wearing rubber bands. If you have teens, you know how difficult it can be to get any information out of them.

Our main treatment area, complete with floor-to-ceiling glass, looks out over a peaceful garden with water features and our famous turtles. These Zen-inducing views are visible from all the chairs in that room, which beats staring at a wall.

We want people to feel as comfortable as if they were coming over to our house for dinner, which is why we have invested in a play area for children, a coffee bar where you can fix yourself a warm beverage, and an area where people can brush their teeth before their appointment.

Over the years, our patients have also grown quite attached to our turtles—a tradition that began with the orthodontist who preceded me. Previous patients who had a pet turtle and decided they could no longer keep it brought it to our office instead of turning it loose. They knew their turtle would be safe and cared for in our office. They also knew that by donating him to our office, they could always visit him anytime they liked.

Everyone, young and old, seems to enjoy watching our turtles (now plural) meander around our turtle habitat. Over the years, they have reproduced, so we also keep the hatchlings in a tank in our reception area for people to see.

WHAT SHOULD I LOOK FOR IN AN INITIAL EVALUATION?

After your tour, one of my assistants will take photos of your face and your teeth. Why do we need to do this? Because the photos are an important record of your initial condition, and we will use this initial impression to formulate a proper diagnosis. Just like physicians need X-rays, MRIs, and lab work to get as complete a picture of what is going on with their patients' bodies as possible, we need the same degree of insight in order to make proper recommendations.

We generally take a panoramic, or full mouth X-ray, unless we have received a copy from your dentist, or unless you are pregnant. We get a wealth of information from this X-ray. We can see if there are missing teeth, extra teeth, root canals, signs of gum disease, or problems with the jaw joints. The X-ray is also used to evaluate the root structure. By examining your dental records and these X-rays, I can begin to create a more formal treatment plan. It either confirms my initial plan or allows me to zero-in on some things that I need to pay closer attention to.

Now it's time to meet your orthodontist. Through conversations with patients, I seek to understand why exactly they have come to my office. Do they have specific concerns about their teeth, smile, or bite? Or have they come to see me because a dentist suggested it? Whatever the case, we want to make sure all concerns are addressed during that first visit.

My exams go beyond just checking your teeth. I begin my examination by looking at your face, carefully studying its proportions, symmetry, and the position of your front teeth, both at rest and when you smile. Orthodontic treatment can influence a person's appearance. It can dramatically improve the symmetry of your face and your smile. And conversely, if done improperly, it can exaggerate existing irregularities.

An examination of your temporomandibular joints (TMJ) and jaw muscles is done to check for any signs of TMJ problems. Clicking or popping of the jaw joint is a sign of a potential problem with your jaw joint. If it's not painful, then it usually doesn't require treatment, but it's important to note its presence. In some cases, it's a good idea to treat a TMJ problem prior to performing orthodontic treatments.

Finally, we turn our attention to your the teeth. I make note of which teeth are present, if there is crowding or spacing, and the relationship between your teeth when you bite down. There is a lot more to orthodontics than simply lining your teeth up. An accurate initial diagnosis can ensure that a proper treatment plan is completed.

When my evaluation is over, we will discuss treatment options. It's important to remember that there is often more than one treatment option available to you, which can range from limited treatments with a removable appliance to full braces and jaw surgery. This is another reason why it's important for you to communicate to your orthodontist what it is that you specifically want to gain from treatment.

Top-Ten Questions to Ask Your Orthodontist on Your First Visit

1. How long have you been an orthodontist?
2. Are you board certified by the American Board of Orthodontics?
3. What type of retainers do you use?
4. How many Invisalign treatments have you completed?
5. How do you handle emergencies?
6. What is included in your fee?
7. What are your hours?
8. Do you use digital or film-based x-rays?
9. Do you have before-and-after examples of cases like mine?
10. Am I allowed in the treatment area with my child?

PAYMENT OPTIONS AND FLEXIBLE FINANCING

Finally, we come to the topic that people dread most of all: "How much is this all going to cost?"

I realize that dental insurance can be very confusing, especially in regards to whether your doctor will accept your insurance or not and how much it will cover. It's important to realize, from the very start, that your dental insurance will not cover the entire amount of your treatment. There are some insurances with participating doctors who have agreed to discount their fees in exchange for being providers.

There may not be, however, a participating provider in your area. If that is the case, then it's possible for your out-of-network benefits to become available. Whatever the case, you should think of your insurance as a discount coupon. Although you may want to use your coupon, you might have to ask yourself whether it's worth cashing in your coupon only to endure shoddy treatment and poor service. In most cases, such trade-offs prove more expensive in the long run.

At our office, we hire financial coordinators whose sole job is to make paying for orthodontic treatment as easy and convenient as possible. We offer several payment options for treatments, such as paying in full with a discount or in-house financing with a down payment. Monthly payments over the course of your treatment or financing from an outside finance company are other possibilities. In the end, we want to make it easy for you to get that million-dollar smile without busting your budget.

If you are comfortable with the doctor and treatment plan, then your treatment can usually begin right away. We will scan your teeth to make digital models, take another quick X-ray, and then you'll be on your way to a confident, beautiful smile and a healthy bite.

GETTING A SECOND OPINION

I realize that orthodontic treatments can be a major investment, which is why you should be wary of any orthodontist who balks at the prospect of you getting a second opinion. It is never unreasonable—under any circumstance—to get more than one opinion on your teeth. Most people get second opinions to compare prices. There's nothing wrong with doing a little comparative shopping, as I realize that we're not all as flush with cash as Bill Gates.

It is never unreasonable—under any circumstance—to get more than one opinion on your teeth.

However, many patients become confused because they get different treatment plans from different doctors. I know that the question most people want to ask is very simple and straightforward, i.e. "My child has crooked teeth. He needs braces. How much?" The problem is that there are many different ways to treat a malocclusion—options that depend on a doctor's level of experience and training. There are, for example, more than a dozen ways to correct an "overbite." Some doctors prefer to remove permanent teeth if there is significant crowding, while others prefer to expand a patient's arches. Some doctors feel that a combination of braces and jaw surgery is the best way to treat certain problems.

Is one undeniably right and the others wrong? No. That's the nature of orthodontics. It's not an exact science, and that's why there are so many options from doctors when it comes to how to treat an orthodontic problem.

What I do ask you to keep in mind is how thorough the orthodontic exam is. The orthodontist should do more than a quick look at the teeth, ask you to "bite down," and say, "Yeah, you need braces." I think you deserve more attention than that.

After undergoing one of my exams and being seen by other doctors, I've had countless people come back to me and remark how much more thorough my exams are than others. I take that as a point of pride—as should you, if you take the time to find the best orthodontist for your particular needs.

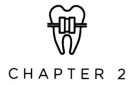

ORTHODONTICS 101: WHAT WE DO AND WHY WE DO IT

Hello, Dear Reader! Chapter 2 explores:

- ◻ *What Is a Proper Bite?*
- ◻ *How Do Teeth Move?*
- ◻ *What an Orthodontist Looks for in an Initial Evaluation*
- ◻ *X-rays, Lasers, and Scanners: A Quick Primer*
- ◻ *What's Really Happening When Appliances Straighten Teeth?*
- ◻ *A Brief History of Orthodontics*

Health care is—or at least *should* be—a service industry. Patients need to be appreciated. And their trust must be earned.

As previously noted, I believe that taking the time to explain fully what will occur during treatment is a major priority in our office.

At the same time, I believe in being respectful of my patients' schedules, which is why we do our best to offer hours that work with their schedules, as opposed to the hours that *I* prefer to work.

I also realize that for most of my patients, time is a precious commodity. They live busy lives and could easily rattle off a dozen other things they'd rather be doing than spending an afternoon in an orthodontist's chair.

Forging long-term relationships with my patients and reaching that critical point where they actually look forward to their next appointment without fear or anxiety is one of the great rewards of my work.

As much as I might long to go into the nitty-gritty details of what I'm doing and why I'm doing it, or talk about the history of orthodontics, I also realize that I have a responsibility to do my work and send my patients back on their way in a reasonable amount of time.

So, consider this chapter to be a condensed primer on orthodontics, which you can glide over—focusing on the bits and pieces you're interested in—or read from start to finish for a more complete education. Feel free to go as deep into the "who," "what," "where," "how," and "why" of orthodontic care as you'd like.

Whatever approach you choose, just know that the following information is what I'd like to tell my patients and parents about orthodontics if we all had the luxury of time.

WHAT IS A PROPER BITE?

In an ideal bite, patients' back teeth should hit evenly when they bite down. The front teeth should just touch lightly. There shouldn't be heavy force weighing down on those. Our jaw isn't just a hinge; it is different from all the rest of the joints in our body in that it is shaped like a U. Instead of simply hinging up and down, our jaw hinges down when first opening, but then the lower jaw essentially slides forward down a slope.

Your jaw can move from side to side, up and down, backward and forward. It goes all over the place. When you bite, the teeth need to mesh together. Every tooth must play its part. Your eyeteeth, for example, are made to guide your posterior teeth apart. Thus, when you're chewing and you make side-to-side motions, you're not wearing the back teeth down excessively. Your jaw muscles learn to close the jaw in the pattern that makes the teeth fit together the best. The way your teeth fit may not be where your jaw joint is fully seated, but this fit will win out in the end, even if it is to the detriment of the jaw joint.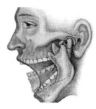

Many people can function just fine with their jaw joints out of position, but it's not a healthy situation. Potentially, problems such as jaw popping, clicking, and joint and facial pain may crop up.

A proper bite includes how the teeth fit together in the back. What we call a class-I occlusion creates a proper relationship of the front teeth, with the upper teeth just in front of the lower teeth so that they work like scissors to cut food. A person with an "overbite" has upper teeth that stick out too far. The opposite problem is an "underbite" where the upper front teeth are trapped behind the lower front teeth, like a bulldog. A class-I occlusion is our goal in most cases because this results in teeth that not only look the best but also function the best.

The way your teeth fit together in the back may be perfect, but the teeth may be too protrusive (meaning they stick out too much). This can occur when a patient's upper and lower front teeth lean too far from the base of their jaw. There is simply too much tooth for the size of the mouth and jaws.

We describe this condition as being able to eat corn through a picket fence. The teeth stick out so much that the person can't comfortably close his or her lips. The teeth may be straight, but they certainly aren't attractive. Patients can be genetically predisposed to have teeth jut out like this, but this protrusion of the teeth can also be created by poorly planned orthodontic treatment.

In young, growing people, our goal is an ideal class-I occlusion. We feel that this is the best for the health, longevity, and appearance of the teeth. In adults, if they have lived with a particular bite all their lives, a "compromise treatment" may be the best way to go. It may be possible to achieve an ideal result, but it would involve jaw surgery and years of treatment when the only thing that bothers the person may be that his or her front teeth are crooked. If the front teeth can be straightened and there are no risks to the health of the teeth, then this compromise treatment may be the most appropriate one.

HOW DO TEETH MOVE?

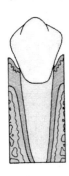

For most of my patients, it's difficult to understand how their teeth—which seem so firmly rooted in their gums—can be altered so dramatically by simple devices like braces and Invisalign trays.

Part of the confusion comes from a basic misunderstanding about teeth in general. Most people tend to think that teeth are directly attached to the bone in their gums, but that's simply not true. There is a small space between the root and the bone that is made up of tiny fibers, blood vessels, nerves, and fluid—a space called the *periodontal ligament*.

Our teeth sit—like kings on a throne—in this pocket of fibers. This band of fibers acts like a shock absorber between your teeth and the bones in your mouth.

Bone is not a static organ. Our bodies are constantly resorbing and depositing bone. It is dissolved and rebuilt constantly, and it happens more in response to the application of force, such as from the pull of muscles.

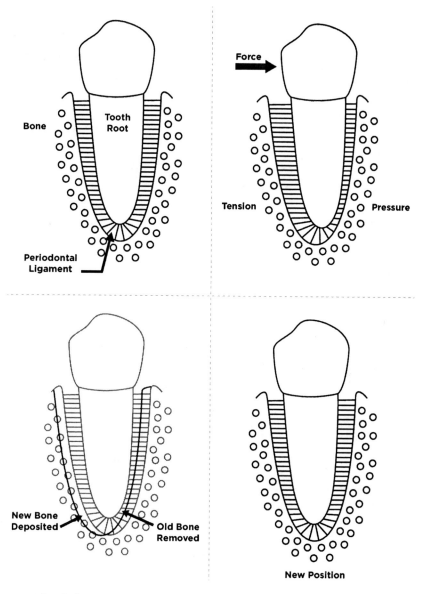

Think for a moment about our elderly population and how often doctors recommend that they stay active in their later years. Exercise is critical for seniors' bone health because the strain of muscles acting on their bones causes more bone to be deposited, thus reducing the risk of osteoporosis.

The bones in your teeth respond to "force" in much the same way. When pressure is applied to one side of your teeth, the bone is removed on the pressure side, and your body lays down bone on the opposite side of that force. Orthodontists know how to apply forces to teeth to achieve the desired movements.

WHAT AN ORTHODONTIST LOOKS FOR DURING AN INITIAL EXAMINATION

It surprises most of my patients to learn that the first thing I look at when performing an initial examination is not my patient's teeth. The first thing I analyze is my patient's *face*. I'm looking, most critically of all, at *proportionality*.

Is your face short or long? Are there any significant asymmetries? (Don't worry; hardly anyone's face is perfectly symmetrical.) I'm looking for any cants to the face or jaws. I'm looking at how much of your upper teeth is displayed when your lips are at rest and when you smile. I'm looking to see if you show any gum tissue when you smile. I also examine the position of your lips. Do your lips close comfortably over the teeth or are they trapped behind teeth that are protruding outward?

All these little details act as critical aids in choosing the best treatment solution for you. It takes more than straight teeth to make a nice smile. A good orthodontist takes all the factors into consideration.

The rest of my examination generally revolves around checking the health and position of your jaw joints (including looking for TMJ problems) and, finally, looking at your teeth and how you bite.

By combining what I learn during my examination with the results of my X-rays, I can accurately map out the best treatment options.

But the final thought I'd like to leave you with is that orthodontics is truly a team sport. Orthodontic work isn't something that's done to a patient. It's done *with* a patient.

It requires substantial effort on the part of the orthodontist and his office team as well as the patient—and, if applicable, parents as well. If everyone does his part, then treatments will progress in a timely manner. If someone doesn't do his job, there tends to be disappointment all around. The orthodontist's role is clear: We're here to properly diagnose the problems and offer appropriate treatment options that will satisfy both our patients' needs and desires in a way that is as convenient and comfortable as possible.

Our teams do their part too. They are an extension of the doctor. They do a lot of the routine work on the patient, such as removing the orthodontic wires at each visit. They evaluate the patient's hygiene, and if it's lacking, they go over how to clean the teeth and braces again. They communicate with the patient and parents, asking if there are any problems or concerns. Many times, the patient is more willing to talk to the assistant about any concerns than with the doctor. The assistants make sure that proper instructions are provided so that patients know exactly what is expected of them. At the end of the appointment, they tell the parent what was done at the visit, how the treatment is progressing, and what is planned for the next visit. Well-trained, talented assistants, working with a doctor who knows how to use their talents, create a fine-tuned machine that can see many patients in an efficient manner.

My patients also play a critical role in successful outcomes. Cooperative patients will have shorter treatment times, superior results, and less chance of problems. For example, cooperation means they keep their teeth clean, they don't break their bands and brackets by eating the wrong foods, and they wear their elastics (rubber bands) or aligners as directed. Patients are also responsible for coming in for their appointments on a regular basis. After a certain amount of time, the braces no longer put force on the teeth, and the teeth stop moving. I've seen patients who haven't been in the office for six months or more come to me and say, "When am I getting these braces off? I've had them on for two years already." The problem is that they can't count that six-month vacation as part of the treatment. I tell them that they can sit in a car, but unless the engine is turned on and someone is driving, they're not going anywhere.

X-RAYS, LASERS, AND SCANNERS: A QUICK PRIMER

During a visit to my office, you are likely to encounter a few orthodontic tools and technologies that may look downright alien to you. Allow me to give you a short introduction to each of these technologies and explain why I have made considerable financial investments in bringing them into our office.

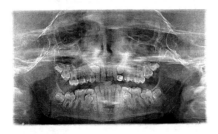

Digital Panoramic X-Ray: Up until the beginning of the 2000s, pretty much all of us—dentists and orthodontists alike—took traditional film X-rays. We snapped a picture of your teeth, developed the film in a darkroom, and then put them up on a light board. We interpreted them and then reported our findings.

In recent years, both myself and other forward-thinking orthodontists have invested in digital X-rays, which use a sensor to scan your mouth and then, in mere seconds, transfer that image onto a computer. There are several advantages to using digital X-rays, including the fact that they are faster, easier for patients to see, and expose you to approximately half the amount of radiation of traditional X-rays.

If your orthodontist is still using film, you should wonder what other outdated techniques he or she might be using.

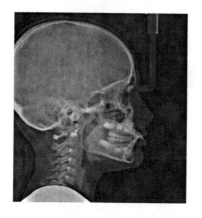

Lateral Cephalogram: The lateral cephalogram, or "**lateral ceph**," is basically just an X-ray of the side of your head with your teeth biting together. Generally, the X-ray is taken from the right side of your face, but occasionally we'll also do one directly head-on, eyes forward, should there be significant facial asymmetries. We use these images to look at the relationship and the position of your jaw relative to your teeth and the rest of your face.

Cone-Beam Technologies: Traditional dental X-rays are no different than the X-rays that your doctor will take, should you break a bone. They are completely two-dimensional. But cone-beam scanners are the orthodontic equivalent of a CAT scan, providing us the ability to capture the structures of your mouth in three dimensions.

By using these three-dimensional images, I can examine your teeth in stunning detail and see exactly where teeth that are not yet in the mouth are positioned. This is very important for impacted teeth, which are teeth that have not erupted—i.e., come in—for one reason or another. In the past, we used to take X-rays and estimate where a tooth was hiding. This could be both bloody and painful, as oral surgeons often had to make a large opening and go searching. With cone-beam scanners, no guesswork is needed. We know exactly where the tooth is located and how to bring it into the mouth—saving you time, money, and discomfort.

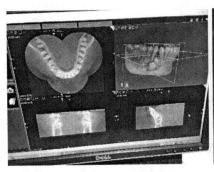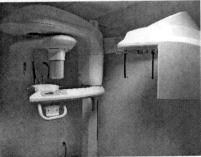

Soft-Tissue Lasers: These miniature lasers are no bigger than your average pen in size, but they can be extraordinarily useful. A fiber-optic cable connects the laser to an energy source, which enables the tip of the device to emit a targeted laser beam.

This laser does not affect either bone or teeth when applied to a patient's mouth. It only impacts soft tissue—specifically, your gums. The doctor gently touches the tip of the laser to the tissue, and it disappears. It gently takes off excess tissue, one tiny layer at a time. In this way, a tooth that is slow to come in can be uncovered, or puffy swollen gums can be recontoured.

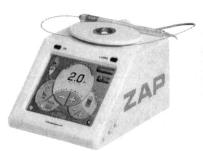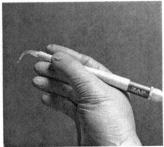

The advantages of using soft-tissue lasers can be profound. Often, we only have to apply a topical anesthetic to numb the area where we are working, thus avoiding the need to use needles. There are no scalpels or stitching of any kind, very little or no bleeding, and very little discomfort afterward. All this can be accomplished by your orthodontist, avoiding the extra time and expense of having to visit another specialist.

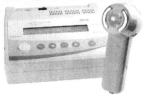

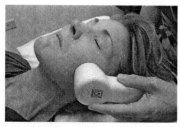

Cold Lasers: Unlike a soft-tissue laser, cold lasers are used to penetrate tissues and help lessen inflammation, especially those linked to TMJ problems and headaches. In addition, it can also be used to reduce discomfort from orthodontic adjustments. Shaped like handheld percussion massagers, cold lasers are applied directly to the skin of a patient's face for several minutes. The cold laser can make orthodontic treatment much more comfortable.

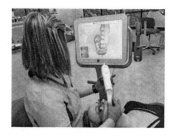

Intraoral Scanner: Before the advent of these scanners, orthodontists had to take molds of patients' teeth: one for the upper jaw and one for the lower. This was necessary to see what a patient's bite looked like and to craft various orthodontic appliances. We tended to use a material called alginate.

When mixed with a liquid, this alginate powder turned into a material similar in consistency to mashed potatoes. This was loaded into a dental tray and placed over the teeth. Patients had to sit in a chair with a mouth filled with this material, which was often uncomfortable. People with a sensitive gag reflex have a particularly difficult time with impressions.

Our intraoral scanner, by contrast, uses a wand that scans the teeth. It takes a series of three-dimensional pictures. Then the computer combines this information and makes a digital model of your teeth. That model can then be sent electronically to laboratories across the country, where they can make whatever appliances, including Invisalign trays, that are required.

In addition, intraoral scanners allow me to look on my computer and see three-dimensional models of your teeth, which can further aid me in my diagnosis. I can see where teeth meet each other and can analyze how much space there is between each tooth, while performing precise measurements on my computer. There is a great number of orthodontists who still abide by the old plaster-model approach. It's comfortable and familiar to them, and they hesitate to make capital investments in a scanner. "Why spend the money on an expensive scanner," they say, "when there's nothing wrong with our plaster models?" Unfortunately, this kind of thinking doesn't consider the comfort of the *patient*.

WHAT'S REALLY HAPPENING WHEN APPLIANCES STRAIGHTEN TEETH?

Say, for example, we use Invisalign trays (we call them aligners) to apply force to the crown of one of your teeth with the intent of moving it toward your lips. The bone on the side of your lips is going to be resorbed, or removed by your body. Then on the tongue side of your mouth, bone will be deposited, allowing your teeth to move.

This straightening occurs because the constant force applied to your teeth is felt by the ligament, which in turn transmits that force to the bone. It's a domino effect. The bone via the ligament is sensing pressure, so it responds in kind by remodeling—adding or subtracting bone—which allows the tooth to move and, if it's moving in the right direction, become straight.

The key, of course, is that the force being applied to your teeth is both gentle and constant. Your teeth are made to resist heavy, intermittent forces that come from chewing. Your periodontal ligament, that aforementioned "throne" in which your individual teeth sit, is made up of fibers and fluids that resist the force of the chewing.

By biting hard for just a second or two, that hydraulic pressure prevents the tooth from moving too much. But if you maintain a constant force, especially if it's a lower force, you start to get the ligament to compress. It slowly squeezes the fluid out. And that's when you start to get noticeable tooth movement.

Apply too much force, and you'll end up crushing your ligament. You'll kill the cells that are resorbing and depositing the bone. That's why I strongly urge patients to see skilled orthodontists instead of practitioners with little or no experience and training. It takes a great deal of experience to know how to apply the right pressure. This is a major misconception among both laypeople and many of my dental colleagues. I'll hear people say, "Go ahead and crank it up, Doc; I want to get done and get these things off." They don't realize that high forces move teeth slower, are more painful, and increase the risk of problems like root resorption. The body responds better to light, continuous force, which stimulates your cells to make proper changes to your bones.

If an appliance is attached to your teeth and not removable by the patient, then it's easier to apply the constant force. If it's a removable appliance, then we rely on the patient to wear the appliance long enough to make the teeth move. Remember, a low, *constant* force is best. An appliance that is just worn while sleeping will not efficiently move teeth. A removable appliance that is not worn an adequate amount of time will only make the teeth get loose, become more sore, and not straighten out.

The point to remember is that these corrections can be performed on teens and adults, even older adults, and yield dramatic benefits.

"Mae," one of my patients, was an older woman, a schoolteacher, who had always hated the way her teeth looked. She was, in fact, so self-conscious of her teeth, she hardly ever smiled. Thus, her students (not to mention other adults) thought she was a stern, grumpy person, even though she was warm and friendly. At some point, she decided she'd had enough and that it was time to do something about it.

As a teacher, having traditional braces was not going to be an option, but with the availability of Invisalign, she figured she could straighten her teeth discretely. She underwent treatment with Invisalign aligners, did great, and now has a beautiful smile that she's not afraid to show. Mae, who never used to smile, now smiles all the time. For several months after her treatment, whenever I would run into her husband, he would just go on and on about the change in his wife. She truly blossomed. People like Mae are the reason that I have the best job in the world.

A Brief History of Orthodontics

The field of orthodontics is a time-tested medical discipline that stretches back more than one hundred years. A dentist named Edward H. Angle is credited with being the father of modern orthodontics, as he focused his practice on the correction and alignment of teeth—and even started the first set of schools to train dentists on how to do orthodontic treatment.

In Dr. Angle's time, braces were very expensive. They were made of gold and custom-fitted with bands around each tooth. For much of the nineteenth and early twentieth centuries, only the very affluent could afford orthodontic treatment.

Even as recently as the 1960s, orthodontic treatments remained expensive, often costing as much as a new car. These prices were the result of the amount of work it took to custom make and fit bands on each tooth. It often took most of a day to place braces on a patient. In addition, most of the work was done by the orthodontist himself. Obviously, this limited how many people could be seen.

Two important developments in the 1970s and 1980s helped make orthodontic treatment more affordable. One was the creation of "preformed" orthodontic bands. Instead of having to create customized bands for each tooth in a patient's mouth, manufacturers began producing preformed bands that could be fitted to a person's teeth and then cemented in place, saving much time and energy. In addition, the advent of dental assistants as a viable profession allowed orthodontists to see more patients per day, bringing the cost of orthodontic treatment within reach for millions of American families.

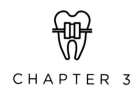

THE ANATOMY OF A SMILE: FINDING YOUR INNER PEARLY WHITES

Hello, Dear Reader! Chapter 3 explores:

- *What Goes into a Nice Smile?*
- *Positioned for Success: How an Orthodontist Achieves Proper Teeth Alignment*
- *Elwood's Story: You're Never Too Old for Orthodontic Treatment*
- *Wisdom about Wisdom Teeth*
- *The Trigonometry of Orthodontics: Odd Angles and Diagonal Teeth*

Whether we like to admit it or not, it's an undeniable fact of life that people tend to make snap judgments about others based on their appearance. We're only human, which means we're not immune to occasionally judging a book by its cover.

Individuals with distinctive facial features have always been easy targets for those looking to belittle others. Look at caricatures and political cartoons. What do you see? Artists who want to make someone to look unintelligent or untrustworthy tend to focus their attention on altering a subject's face, often by doctoring his or her smile into a gummy grin or gapped buck teeth that would give Bugs Bunny pause.

The truth of the matter is that smiles matter. Numerous research studies have analyzed how people react to certain facial structures and smiles. Show a random group of people photos of individuals with unattractive smiles or awkward-looking teeth and they'll almost invariably perceive them to be unintelligent, unsophisticated, or even dishonest.

Show those same groups images of the same subjects, only this time with corrected smiles, and they'll view them in a far more favorable light.

And it's precisely for this reason that I tell my patients that orthodontic work is one of the best overall values in health care, as it doesn't just offer physiological benefits but psychological ones as well!

Children with protruding or extremely crooked teeth are particularly prone to be misjudged, not only by their peers but also by teachers and coaches. The effects of these judgments can be crippling for children.

Bullies find children with unusual-looking teeth to be easy marks and often begin to inflict psychological and emotional pain at an early age. Taunts and teasing cause a ripple effect. When children are treated as if they are unintelligent, their performance often dips to reflect that image.

Nor does the bullying stop there. Teenagers and adults with unflattering smiles face equally complex challenges. When two people are applying for a job with the same credentials, one with crooked teeth and the other with a smile like George Clooney, which one do you think is going to get the job?

There has been ample research showing that people with unattractive smiles pay the price of these judgments in terms of career opportunities and social standing. Being able to flash an attractive smile isn't, therefore, just an aesthetic advantage. Research shows that people with bad teeth who are competing for jobs, respect, and romantic partners are working with a serious handicap.

WHAT GOES INTO A NICE SMILE?

There's no getting around the fact that most of my patients come to see me for aesthetic reasons, not for health emergencies. They realize the importance of a nice smile and proportional facial features and are committed to undergoing orthodontic treatments to correct them.

What most of my patients don't realize is that there is a great deal more involved with achieving a nice smile than simply straightening their front teeth. While it's often difficult for them to pinpoint what exactly is irregular about their teeth, they know, on an almost instinctual level, that something is a bit off. What they need is someone with more experienced eyes to identify the issue.

As orthodontists, we're trained to see—and fix—the multitude of variables that go into generating a beautiful smile. You can have straight teeth, for example, but if an excessive amount of gum tissue comes peeking out every time you smile, it's not going to register as attractive to others.

I bring up the example of "gummy smiles" because they can be the result of a range of factors, most of which are impossible for an average patient to identify.

First, they can arise due to something we call "over-erupted teeth," which means your teeth have actually grown too much. If you have over-erupted teeth, the supporting structures of your gums and bones have grown out too far from your jaw. Your top teeth are growing too far downward and your bottom teeth are growing too far upward.

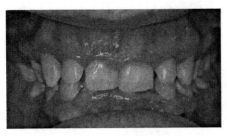

Short upper front teeth due to wear.

Second, a gummy smile can be due to teeth that have worn down over time and, therefore, have over-erupted, revealing more of your gums when you smile. These teeth tend to be short and square. In extreme cases, they are wider than they are long.

A gummy smile can also emerge when gum tissue covers too much of your teeth. You have normally shaped teeth, but half of them is covered by the gums. This is a condition that often self-corrects as a person enters adulthood, but sometimes it does not, and this must be recognized to be properly treated.

The fourth reason for a gummy smile is hyperactive upper lip muscles. When smiling, the upper lip pulls up too far, exposing all the upper teeth and gums like a window shade that goes too far up.

The point here is that there is so much more going on than just the alignment of your front teeth, and the treatment required to correct these issues will depend on what is wrong.

For example, people with a deep bite can be treated by moving their upper front teeth up, their lower front teeth down, or a combination of the two. The goal is to place the upper front teeth in the proper relationship with the upper lip.

One misconception is that the bone and gums are a static entity and that we only move teeth. The supporting bone and gums are affected according to where the teeth that they support go. A tooth that is moved up doesn't sink into the gums; the bone and gums all go up with the teeth. This is how we can reduce how much gum shows when a person smiles.

In the instance where the teeth are worn down and over-erupted, patients tend to have short square teeth. The dentist can't restore the teeth to a normal length, because when the patient bites down, the teeth hit the opposing teeth and there is no room to make the tooth longer. In this case, the proper treatment is to intrude the teeth (move them up toward the gums), make room, and then have a dentist restore the teeth to their normal lengths.

A young person with too much gum covering his or her teeth due to an overgrowth of gum tissue may not want to wait and see if the condition improves over time. Appearance is very important to the average teenager, and they are often bothered by having little teeth.

Fortunately, they don't need to just "deal with it." A simple surgical procedure to remove excess gum tissue, often using a soft-tissue laser, can correct this problem.

When a gummy smile is the result of hyperactive lip muscles, the solution is to prevent the lip from pulling up too far when smiling. This can be corrected with Botox injections. Unfortunately, it's not a permanent fix and patients often have to go back for periodic reinjections.

POSITIONED FOR SUCCESS: HOW AN ORTHODONTIST ACHIEVES PROPER TEETH ALIGNMENT

I gave this litany of examples regarding gummy smiles to underscore the importance of turning to a skilled orthodontist.

A good orthodontist will take a multitude of factors into consideration, including the gum tissue and the shape of the teeth.

Orthodontists are part of a team that includes a general dentist, periodontist, oral surgeon, and others. Good orthodontists know when additional help is required to produce a truly outstanding result. Remember, to a man with a hammer, every problem is a nail. You want to make sure your doctor is looking at the big picture and not just what falls within their expertise. I have the added experience of having completed a general-practice residency program and having practiced general dentistry for several years before going back to school for orthodontic training. This experience helps me see the big picture as well as a patient's overall dental condition.

Another thing to understand is that there is no single formula for straightening teeth. There is no consensus on what is the best final position of the teeth. Some orthodontists like to finish with broad smiles and others prefer narrower jaws. Maybe one doctor's patients complete treatment with teeth that are straight up and down and others not so much. Unfortunately, a lot of this comes down to what is in fashion and the hottest trend. Most orthodontists try to offer treatments that are supported by good evidence—but, in so many cases, the evidence is just not there, so we go with what our training and experience tells us is best. This is an excellent reason to look at before-and-after photos of cases that are similar to your problem. Does your doctor's plan make sense? Is it something you are comfortable with? For example, have you been told you need permanent teeth removed, or that you need jaw surgery, or a night brace? If you see three different orthodontists, you'll probably leave with three different plans. Go with the one that takes care of your concerns with the doctor that you like and trust.

A good orthodontist can visualize the current position of your teeth, then map out the best and least invasive way to align them into their correct positions. It takes a certain innate ability, but more than anything else, it demands patience, effort, and experience. This is the artsy side of orthodontics. Your orthodontist needs to have some artistic ability, because the final arrangement of your teeth will come down to that.

Thus, proper orthodontic work is both a science and an art. The director of my orthodontic program often said, "Anyone can start an orthodontic case, but very few can finish it."

One area of controversy in orthodontic treatment involves the removal of permanent teeth. There are doctors who recommend removal of permanent teeth frequently and others who proclaim that they never remove teeth. In my office, I don't like to remove teeth unless I am absolutely certain it's the right course of action. I tell my patients, "We can always take them out later, but we can never put them back in." So, sometimes we do what we call "a waffle." We start out by leaving the teeth in place and see how they respond to treatment. Can we, for example, expand your arches enough to align your teeth and generate an attractive smile? If we can't accommodate all the teeth without jeopardizing the health or appearance of the teeth, then we have some removed and use the space to properly position the teeth, closing the space completely.

As unusual as it may sound, teeth that are too straight up and down—i.e., positioned too vertically, like mini chisels—can cause problems as well. Your front teeth should lean forward just a little bit, with your top teeth positioned just in front of your bottom teeth, much like the way the two blades of a scissors overlap.

If you've ever seen someone with sunken-in lips, it could be the result of his or her teeth being too straight up and down. It's also common in elderly patients, because as we age, our noses and chins continue to grow, which allows our lips to recede.

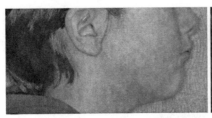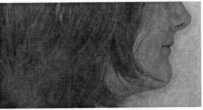

Before and after poor orthodontic treatment.

I've seen this condition in more than one of my patients, including a thirteen-year-old girl who looked like she had the facial structure of a sixty-year-old woman. Her orthodontist removed several permanent teeth, and then the gaps in her mouth were closed by tipping her front teeth backward. The damage was done, and it took two more years of treatment to correct.

Elwood's Story: You're Never Too Old for Orthodontic Treatment

Elwood was a grandfather who had footed the bill for braces for both his children and several of his grandchildren. At some point, he began to think that maybe it was his turn to see an orthodontist. His teeth had always been crooked, but he didn't like the prospect of walking around with braces at his age. Once we talked about Invisalign, he knew he'd found the perfect choice. The Invisalign trays worked perfectly, and now he has a smile he can be proud of, just like his kids and grandkids.

WISDOM ABOUT WISDOM TEETH

Wisdom teeth, which are also called your third molars, have taken too much blame for crooked teeth for far too long! I hear complaints about wisdom teeth constantly, usually from adults who had braces when they were teenagers. Often, they come into my office, point to their wisdom teeth, and grumble about how their teeth used to be perfectly straight until their wisdoms "made them go crooked."

If you look at wisdom teeth on a panoramic X-ray, it's easy to assume that they may be to blame. They look, on film, like they are literally ramming into the teeth in front of them. But in reality, they don't contribute that much to the crowding of your teeth. There is an important study that compared patients with wisdom teeth to patients who were missing them (i.e., their wisdom teeth didn't form). The results were identical: Similar crowding and crookedness occurred whether there were wisdom teeth in place or not.

So why then do some people's teeth go crooked? The honest answer is that we're not 100 percent sure, but we have given the phenomenon a name: *late developmental crowding.* This usually occurs in white populations, so there is probably a genetic component to it. But the good news is that these problems can often be prevented with a proper retainer.

THE TRIGONOMETRY OF ORTHODONTICS: ODD ANGLES AND DIAGONAL TEETH

When I examine a patient's teeth, I'm not only looking at their alignment and position relative to the gums. I'm also looking at the shape of the teeth and how they are angled. Here are some examples of irregularly angled teeth.

Tilted Teeth: Teeth that are angled a little bit too much to one side or another are very noticeable to everyone. This was the problem that Tom Cruise had for many years until he had it corrected. In an ideal world, the center of your teeth should be perfectly aligned with the center of your face, i.e. the "Cupid's Bow" dip in the middle of your upper lip. But if your front teeth are just a bit off-center and your teeth are angled properly, no one will notice the asymmetry.

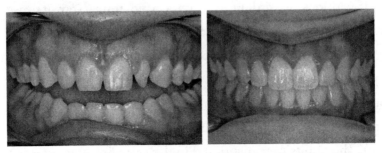

(L) Poorly tapered teeth. (R) Well-shaped teeth.

Irregularly Shaped Teeth: Although there is no clear definition as to what constitutes the perfect shape of a tooth, it's generally agreed that your upper front teeth should be at their widest at their incisal edges (the edges of the teeth that you use to bite into things) and then gradually recede in size toward the gum line. Should your teeth be widest near the gum line and then taper down, this can give the appearance of extra space between your teeth.

The Smile Line: When a person smiles, the edges of his or her upper teeth should follow the curve of the lower lip. They shouldn't go straight across, or heaven forbid, curve in the opposite direction in a clown-like grimace.

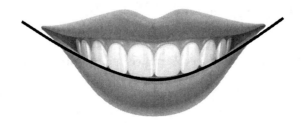

Dark Triangles: Should your teeth be excessively triangular in shape and you find some recession of your gums, you have what we orthodontists call *dark triangles*. Basically, the tips of your teeth touch, but there is a gap between your teeth leading up to the gum lines. If you're young, gum tissue tends to fill in that triangular space, but if you're old and your gums recede, you have a dark shape that looks as dark as the Bermuda Triangle, thus the term dark triangles.

All the above issues are treatable conditions. They can be addressed in various ways, whether it's simply reshaping your teeth by removing a little enamel, altering the shape of your teeth by adding some tooth-colored filling material, or applying veneers (chapter 5 covers veneers). Your orthodontist will work with your general dentist to position the teeth so they can be restored to an optimal shape.

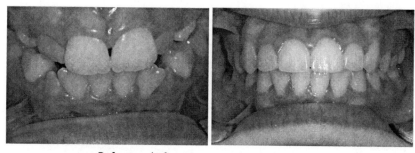

Before and after treatment for dark triangle.

In the end, it's best to remember one thing: Not all orthodontists pay attention to details such as this.

Let me leave you with a cautionary tale: I once saw a teenage girl who began treatments with another orthodontist because of her family's insurance coverage. The girl was missing a permanent upper bicuspid and had the baby tooth in its place. The orthodontist wanted to treat the girl with the removal of four bicuspid teeth: two on the top and two on the bottom. This is not an unusual plan of action. The problem is that when a permanent tooth is missing, it is generally best to remove the baby tooth that's taking the place of the missing permanent tooth and close that space. In this girl's case, a permanent bicuspid was removed instead of the baby tooth.

This treatment, to put it mildly, didn't do this young lady any favors. She had a perfectly good permanent tooth removed instead of removing the baby tooth. Now she is at risk of losing that baby tooth in the future and will be left with the expensive proposition of having it replaced. A word of advice: Cheaper, quicker treatments in the short term might lead to more expensive and painful treatments in the long run.

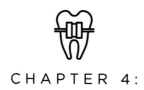

CHAPTER 4:

BRACE YOURSELF: A GUIDE TO BRACES, BRACKETS, AND INVISALIGN

Hello, Dear Reader! Chapter 4 *explores:*

- *Will My Braces Hurt?*

- *Innovations and Aesthetics: A Look at Today's Braces*

- *How Will Braces Affect My Life?*

- *What Is the Damon Bracket?*

- *What Are Rubber Bands for?*

- *What Is Invisalign and What Can It Treat?*

- *Weighing Your Options: The Pros and Cons of Invisalign*

If I can implore you to do one thing as you consider braces, it's to remember this: Today's braces are not your father's braces, and in some cases, they're not even your older sibling's braces.

All those horror stories you might have heard about how painful it is to get braces and how a trip to the orthodontist's office inevitably means you're going to get your teeth yanked out are as outdated as disco music and eight-track tapes.

In the late 1970s and early 1980s, braces were far different, both in terms of discomfort and aesthetics, than they are today. Back then, most braces were still attached to a patient's teeth with awkward, old-fashioned bands.

They were, in essence, mini rings for your teeth: thin metal rings that were adapted to each tooth and cemented in place. Welded to these bands were the orthodontic brackets that held the orthodontic wires in place.

As a result, a great deal of metal was visible, with only a hint of tooth enamel showing. Due to the thickness of these bands and the brackets, braces weren't very comfortable, either. Back then, when an orthodontist removed a patient's braces, little gaps often remained between individual teeth. Patients, therefore, had to wear retainers that could be adjusted to close these "band spaces." In addition, the bulk of these bands meant less space to align the teeth, thus there was a tendency to remove permanent teeth, especially bicuspids.

Thankfully, the days of huge amounts of metal "train tracks" running across people's teeth—not to mention old insults like "metal mouth" or "tin grin"—are pretty much long gone, as the field of orthodontics has made extraordinary strides in terms of aesthetics and comfort in recent years.

WILL MY BRACES HURT?

Let's begin with the question that I most often encounter during initial visits: "How much is this going to hurt?"

The truth is that our procedures in the office are relatively painless, especially in comparison to what most people expect. The teeth will get sore for most people, but it usually occurs some four to six hours after an appointment. It goes without saying that the amount of discomfort varies from person to person. But, generally, it's going to be similar to the soreness you might feel after exercising a muscle for the first time. The next day, your muscles are going to ache when you move them. You can expect the same sort of discomfort when it comes to braces.

Most often, that soreness comes when patients try to bite into and chew their food. Therefore, we recommend very soft foods when your braces are first applied—ideally, foods you can eat with a spoon. Even a peanut butter sandwich made with the softest white bread may be too painful to bite into.

The good news is that the pain associated with braces can often be substantially alleviated by taking the same over-the-counter pain medication you would use for headaches or muscle pains, such as acetaminophen or ibuprofen.

Whatever your pain threshold, it's important to remember that your discomfort will be temporary. Typically, the worst pain comes the day after your braces are placed—then it gets better over the following days. Within a week, most people have become accustomed to their braces.

Your mouth also needs to get used to braces being on the teeth. They will feel huge and foreign at first. (But believe it or not, it feels just as strange when they are removed when the treatment is complete.) You may develop sores on the lips and cheeks from being irritated by the braces.

Fortunately, we offer our patients orthodontic wax, a soft wax that can be molded over the appliances to ease irritation. Should you feel irritation, we recommend that you address it right away to prevent it from becoming a sore or ulcer. After a week or two, your mouth will adjust, and you won't need to use the wax as much, if at all.

If we've treated you with a removable appliance, then you must take time to adjust to it. In the end, it all comes down to the old adage "practice makes perfect." The more you talk with an appliance while it's in place, the sooner you will be able to speak normally. If you're constantly removing the appliance because you can't talk as easily, you will never get used to it, and your treatment times will drag on as a result. Fortunately, children are often much more adaptable than their parents, easily adjusting to changes after a day or two—a valuable lesson to my adult patients.

INNOVATIONS AND AESTHETICS: A LOOK AT TODAY'S BRACES

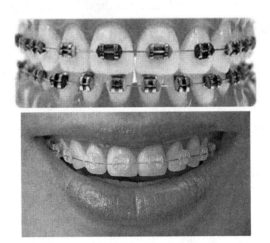

Today, the brackets are directly bonded to the tooth enamel instead of relying on a metal band to hold them in place. Therefore, a relatively small amount of metal is visible. Some orthodontists still use bands, mainly on molars, because these bands are far sturdier and more resistant to being knocked loose when chewing. Beyond that, applying bands is now more of a personal preference. Some orthodontists still choose to use bands on all of a patient's back teeth, while others prefer simply to bond attachments directly to the teeth, showing no interest in using bands at all.

In recent years, we've also seen a greater variety of brackets come onto the market. Some of the most popular are silver-colored stainless-steel braces that we can place "colors" upon. The colors come from colored elastomeric ligatures, which are similar to little rubber bands that hold the wires into the brace. They are removed and new ones are placed during each visit so patients can have fun picking out their colors of choice for the next month.

Many of my patients change colors based on what holidays are on the horizon: pink and red in February; green in March; red, white, and blue in July; black and orange in October; red and green in December. Some of my patients prefer to choose hues that reflect their school colors or the colors of their favorite sports teams. And of course, should a patient want to draw the least attention to the fact that he or she even has braces, there's the option of porcelain brackets, which are basically the same color as the teeth.

HOW WILL BRACES AFFECT MY LIFE?

It would be disingenuous for me to tell you that orthodontic treatments won't, in some way, impact your daily life, but often not in the ways you might expect them to.

Most people, for instance, think that chewing gum is strictly prohibited if they have braces, but in reality, chewing gum (if it's sugarless) rarely causes any problems. Some studies show that it may help with tooth movement—and decrease discomfort.

When it comes to restrictions regarding food, there are really only two macro categories of things to avoid: sticky stuff and hard, crunchy stuff.

The sticky stuff is the type of thing that makes your teeth stick together a bit, like caramel and taffy. Gooey sweets tend to stick to your teeth—and your braces—and can pull them off your teeth. In my experience, the worst offender in the sticky category is undeniably a package of Jolly Ranchers.

No matter how much you may love them, they are to be avoided at all costs. Jolly Ranchers are so pernicious, in fact, there is a dental product designed to remove dental crowns that is basically the same consistency as a Jolly Rancher.

Crunchy things, including cereals, nuts, ice, and corn chips, often prove to be dangerous as well. Basically, I have a simple rule. If it's a snack that ends with an "O," like Doritos, Fritos, and Tostitos, it probably will be on your "don't eat" list.

But some braces-destroying habits are far less obvious. People who nervously gnaw on pens and pencils are virtually guaranteed to do serious damage to their braces, as those actions and motions are very similar to the techniques we use to remove braces in the first place.

Should something happen to your braces, the best advice I can give is to be honest with your orthodontist. I've had patients come to me with broken brackets and swear they were on a strict "mashed potato only" diet. And in some cases, through no fault of their own, their braces really did get damaged.

On the other hand, I've had a fortunate few confess to me that they ate every sticky, crunchy snack they could consume—and their braces remained as undamaged as the day they were applied. The truth is that there are a multitude of factors, including variations in people's enamel, as well as how violently they clench and grind their teeth when they sleep, that can affect how tightly the bond strength of their brackets holds up.

WHAT IS THE DAMON BRACKET?

Several years ago, there was a lot of excitement surrounding what we call "Damon brackets," which differ from traditional braces only in that each bracket has a little "door" that holds the wire in place instead of the colored elastic rubber-band-like ligature.

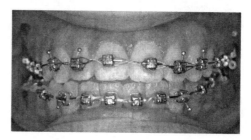

It was theorized that these little doors made each bracket into a "tube" that allowed the orthodontic wires to slide through with less friction, and thus the movement of patients' teeth would occur faster and with less discomfort. However, when research was done comparing Damon brackets to regular brackets, the claims didn't stand up to scrutiny. Teeth weren't corrected more quickly, pain didn't decrease, and you could do everything with regular braces that were claimed by Damon advocates.

There is one advantage, however, to choosing Damon brackets. They are faster to remove and place the orthodontic wires—i.e., the amount time you spend in my chair each visit will decrease.

Why is that? Because when our patients come in to get their braces adjusted, we typically have to take the wires out. Then we either put new wires in or we adjust the existing ones. With traditional braces, each little piece of colored plastic must be taken off so the wires can be removed. Then our patients go brush their teeth, and when they come back, we adjust the wires. After the adjustment, fresh little rubber bands are put back on.

With a Damon bracket, there are no little pieces of plastic to take on and off. We just slide open the doors, take the wires out, put them back in, close the doors, and we're done. Unfortunately, most of my patients with traditional braces are young people who want "colors" on their braces, negating the one advantage of the Damon bracket.

There were, however, some positive developments that resulted from all the excitement over the Damon bracket. Dr. Damon showed that it's possible to properly treat collapsed, crowded arches (even in adults) by using braces and expanding a patient's arches instead of removing teeth. His findings opened the eyes of scores of orthodontists, myself included, and as a result, we can often expand a patient's arches instead of removing teeth to resolve crowding.

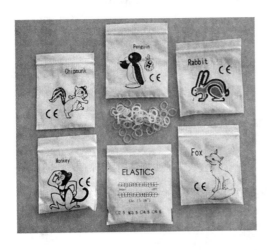

WHAT ARE RUBBER BANDS FOR?

By now, most people are familiar with the rubber bands that we apply to braces. The main reason we apply them is to help correct one's bite. If a person has upper teeth that stick out too far, then rubber bands are worn from the upper front teeth to the lower back molars, pulling the upper teeth back and the lower teeth forward.

The rubber bands, which are smaller than traditional ones, are set in place by the patients themselves and removed to eat and to brush. There are exceptions, but elastics need to be worn pretty much all the time to work properly. That means you have to wear them day and night and only take them out when eating and brushing.

It's a 24/7 responsibility. If you don't wear them as directed, they won't work, and you'll only add months to your treatment time.

Orthodontists can also, by the way, tell whether you are wearing them or not. When you come to your appointments and your bite hasn't changed, we are pretty sure you aren't wearing your elastics properly.

You may wonder why the bags of rubber bands have some animal or memorable name on them. The elastics come in many sizes and strengths. It's easier for a patient to remember that they are wearing, say, "gorillas," than the actual 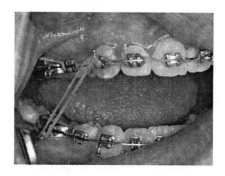 diameter of the elastic, like 5/16th of an inch, or a number that represents how much tension each rubber band has when it's stretched three times its diameter, like five ounces.

WHAT IS INVISALIGN AND WHAT CAN IT TREAT?

The Invisalign appliance is a removable appliance—as opposed to braces, which are glued to the teeth—that straightens the teeth using a number of different "aligners" (our fancy word for the trays). During each stage of an Invisalign treatment, a patient places a new aligner, which straightens the teeth just a little bit at a time.

The easiest way to think about Invisalign is to envision a series of trays, each of which has been customized to adjust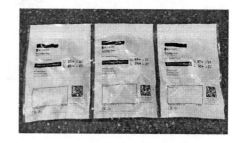

your teeth in subtle but important ways. You're likely to swap out one tray for another every week or two. The number of trays varies per person from five to as many as fifty or more, depending on the severity of your issue. I've found that changing them on a weekly basis usually delivers the best results. In fact, Invisalign has recently modified their recommendation to changing trays every week instead of every two weeks.

I have had my patients change their aligners weekly for the past several years, and our office was part of a study that Invisalign conducted to determine whether weekly changing of aligners was safe and effective.

In addition, I slow down the tooth movement between each aligner, so that they are less tight and restrictive when first put in. This makes the treatment more comfortable and the results more predictable.

With Invisalign, you will need to have attachments placed on certain teeth. The attachments are little "bumps" made of tooth-

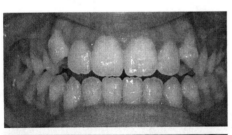
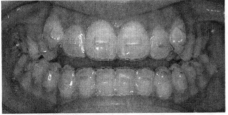

colored filling material. The attachments give the aligners something to push against, which in turn move your teeth. The attachments are a non-negotiable, absolutely necessary part of an effective Invisalign treatment. Don't worry, they are not very noticeable. You will get used to them quickly, and they are a thousand times better than having traditional orthodontic brackets.

Invisalign has invested a great deal of capital in both researching the effectiveness of its products and in constantly developing new and better attachments, which is why Invisalign is the acknowledged leader in the field of clear orthodontic aligners. The materials that can be used for the attachments can vary. Your doctor should use a material that blends with the color of your teeth to make them as inconspicuous as possible.

They will feel, during the early stages of treatment, a bit bulky or foreign—same as with anything new in your mouth—but my patients tend to adjust to them very quickly. When the aligners are being worn (which should be most of the time), you will often forget that they are even there.

In our office, the first two sets of aligners do not have any attachments. Think of them as training wheels. We want you to get used to putting them in and taking them out without the added effort of having to deal with attachments on your teeth.

After two weeks, we have a longer visit when the attachments are added, and then we show patients how to properly put the aligners in and take them out.

It is true that the attachments make placing and removing the trays a bit more challenging, but we teach our patients how to pop them out with relative ease. After a while, it becomes second nature. We also give you a case to put the aligners in while you eat.

When the treatment is complete, the attachments are removed and we polish your teeth.

People can eat freely with their aligners in, provided they do their best to keep them clean and don't consume too many sugary foods. However, most prefer to remove them while eating. It is very important that they be removed when drinking soft drinks and fruit juices. These drinks tend not only to be packed with sugar but are very acidic as well, making them a corrosive one-two combination for any kind of orthodontic treatment. Citrus juices, especially, should be avoided, as they are the equivalent of battery acid for your teeth and can do serious damage if left in contact with your enamel for very long. They will dissolve your teeth.

One thing that my patients sometimes notice with Invisalign aligners is that their bite sometimes will feel a little "off" when the aligners are not in their mouth. The thickness of the plastic between one's teeth can create small gaps. It's nothing to worry about, however, as the small gaps are just temporary. By the time your treatment is complete, all your teeth should touch evenly.

Sometimes the orthodontist will ask you to wear elastics, or "rubber bands," with your aligners. This is usually done to correct your bite, either shifting the top teeth back or the lower teeth forward to correct an "overbite" or an "underbite." The elastics can be worn

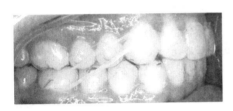

from notches in the aligners or small "buttons" that are applied directly to the teeth, like the attachments we discussed earlier.

The last thing you need to know about Invisalign treatment is that there can be extraordinary differences in the skill levels of dentists and orthodontists when it comes to using Invisalign. It's not uncommon to find a general dentist who has had no more than a few hours of training in orthodontics or a university-trained orthodontist who has rarely worked with the products.

The Invisalign website has a doctor-locator to help you find doctors in your area. Be careful, though; both general dentists and orthodontists are included in the list, unless you specifically choose to search for orthodontists only. Next, the doctors are ranked according to their experience. But be warned: Anyone who is less than an elite doctor is a dabbler, and unless your case is very simple, he or she is going to steer you toward traditional braces.

Should you choose to go with Invisalign, I strongly encourage you to ask your provider questions about his or her experience. In the United States, the average orthodontist spends 80 percent of his or her time working with traditional braces, while only 20 percent with Invisalign. They limit the patients they treat with Invisalign to only the simplest of cases. If you are interested in Invisalign treatment, your doctor's experience will make a big difference.

In my practice, for example, I offer Invisalign to all my full-treatment cases, and more than 60 percent of those patients choose Invisalign. I've used traditional braces for decades, but I've also dedicated hundreds of hours of continuing education to Invisalign since 2002. This experience and education allows me to be confident in working with both approaches.

It's human nature to want to stay in one's comfort zone, and for most orthodontists their comfort zone remains traditional braces. Unless a case is simple and straightforward, they are going to steer people toward traditional braces rather than Invisalign, despite the desires of their patients.

Who is a good candidate for Invisalign? It's not always who you would expect. Let me give you an example about a young patient named Ryan, a boy I'd known since he was just a few years old.

I had treated his mom, and she'd brought Ryan to her appointments where he would play with whatever truck he found in our play area. When Ryan was twelve, he was finally ready for braces. I told his mom that he could be treated with traditional braces or Invisalign. At first, Mom said that braces are kind of a rite of passage for teenagers, so he should go with traditional braces. But then a friend told her about the benefits of Invisalign treatment over traditional braces—and about how great her own daughter was doing—so Ryan's mom decided to try Invisalign for her son. Despite being a fun-loving rascal—an all-American boy—Ryan did great wearing his trays and ended up with an outstanding result. In fact, I submitted his case to Invisalign and he was chosen as one of the top one hundred cases in 2014.

WEIGHING YOUR OPTIONS: THE PROS AND CONS OF INVISALIGN

The truth is that there is a host of misconceptions about Invisalign floating around, both in the general public and the dental profession as well.

Invisalign is *not*, for example, a treatment reserved only for adults or for minor orthodontic problems. It isn't more expensive than traditional braces nor does it demand that all your permanent teeth be erupted. And Invisalign certainly doesn't take longer to correct your teeth than traditional braces.

In 2000, when Invisalign was first introduced, it may have fallen short of what traditional braces could offer, but today I offer Invisalign to all my patients, precisely because for many people, it is the superior choice.

In some cases, Invisalign corrects teeth faster than traditional braces. In addition, there are no diet restrictions involved with Invisalign treatments, as long as the trays are removed when eating. Doritos and Tostitos are, in other words, fair game.

Patients who choose Invisalign simply clean their teeth by removing their trays and brushing and flossing as they would normally. There are no swollen, puffy gums at the end of treatment. Discomfort is rarely a concern as the forces on the teeth are more gentle and controlled and there are no wires poking your mouth. No loose bands or brackets. And no orthodontic emergencies.

For those playing sports, it's easier to wear a mouth guard; for musicians, it's more comfortable to play wind instruments.

Invisalign aligners are changed weekly before going to bed. The aligners tend to feel a little tight when first put in, but by morning they feel fine.

It is also important to note that one of the auxiliary benefits of using Invisalign is that it sometimes helps patients who want to shed a few pounds lose weight.

In one case, I watched one of my patients, a young teacher, drop more than thirty pounds simply because Invisalign provided him the willpower to stop snacking. He told me that he could finally resist the cookies, snacks, and other treats that often found their way into his teachers' lounge, because he didn't want to go through the hassle of removing his aligners every afternoon. With that in mind, Invisalign may also motivate you to drink more water instead of sodas and sweet beverages, thus helping trim your waistline along with reducing your sugar intake.

The Truth About Invisalign

Common Myths that Are Untrue

- Only for adults
- Only for minor orthodontic problems
- More expensive than traditional braces
- Takes longer than traditional braces

- All permanent teeth need to be erupted
- It doesn't work

Advantages of Invisalign over Traditional Braces

- Less noticeable
- No diet restrictions
- Easy to brush and floss
- Easier to wear an athletic mouth guard
- Easier to play wind instruments
- No broken brackets or wire-poke emergencies
- Short, easy appointments
- Fewer visits to the orthodontist
- Less discomfort
- Healthier gums
- Less chance of root resorption (excessive shortening of tooth roots)
- Similar treatment time
- Similar cost
- Equal results

THE GREAT DEBATE: INVISALIGN VS. TRADITIONAL BRACES

In surveying these advantages, choosing Invisalign might sound, in the words of some of my patients, like a "no-brainer." But over the years, I've found that there are two reasons why some people still prefer traditional braces over Invisalign. First and foremost, some patients simply don't have the discipline to wear their Invisalign trays regularly enough for them to work efficiently. Ideally, they should be worn twenty-two hours per day and only taken out during meals and when brushing your teeth.

Invisalign simply doesn't work well for people who snack constantly, nor for people who are absent-minded.

The other reason why some patients, especially young girls, choose traditional braces is because they can create customized "looks" with the "colors." If they have friends with braces with colors, then that's what they want as well. They want to be like their friends—and it doesn't matter how superior another choice may be (the old "if your friend jumped off a bridge…").

In these cases, I usually recommend to parents that they don't fight too hard against their children's wishes, because their cooperation is crucial to the success of the treatment. If they aren't on board with the treatment choice, it's going to be disappointing for everyone. The truth is that some kids are willing to make grand sacrifices for the sake of style or being able to make a personal fashion statement, even if it's with their braces.

I wish I could tell you that there was some simple test I could administer that would tell me if a patient was more suited for Invisalign or traditional braces, but I haven't devised one yet. Some people who come into my office seem like they would be great Invisalign patients but wind up being ill-suited for the task. And then there are others—a few teenage boys come to mind—who I assume will never have the discipline for Invisalign, yet wind up doing perfectly.

One thing is for certain: Gender doesn't play a role when it comes to the success of Invisalign. My female patients are not necessarily better-suited than the males. I have plenty of nice young ladies who don't wear their aligners and don't brush their teeth, and young men who are superstars. One thing that I have noticed is that young patients, those who are eleven, twelve, or in their early teens, seem to do better than "responsible" adults.

I believe this is true because young patients tend to adjust to new things easier and tend to follow their doctors' orders.

Faster, Faster, Faster: What Are Accelerated Orthodontic Treatments?

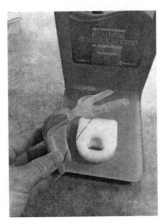

The hottest new trend in orthodontics is something we call "accelerated orthodontic treatment." Who, after all, wouldn't want to get their braces off in one year instead of two? There are several ways to speed up tooth movement, but they generally fall into one of two categories: invasive and non-invasive.

Invasive measures involve doing some form of guided trauma to the bone around the teeth. This creates what is called a regional acceleratory phenomenon, or RAP effect. It increases the number of cells that resorb and deposit bone. This RAP effect can be achieved with full-mouth periodontal surgery called Wilkodontics, which was named after the Wilko brothers that developed the technique.

We can induce a RAP effect without the cost and discomfort of full-mouth surgery by doing micro perforations—small holes made in the bone adjacent to the teeth that we want to move quicker. "Propel" is the product that is used for making the micro perforations. This technique is particularly valuable for speeding up tooth movement in specific areas, such as closing a space for a missing tooth.

Non-invasive treatments, on the other hand, don't require any numbing or traumatic procedures. An AcceleDent device is a mouthpiece that is held between the teeth for twenty minutes per day, which produces a low-level vibration that speeds up tooth movement. This is used to decrease the overall treatment time of the teeth. The good news for all patients is that the AcceleDent device can be used with traditional braces or Invisalign and can sometimes cut the treatment time in half while reducing soreness. I'm proud to say that we use both the Propel and AcceleDent techniques in our office and have had great success.

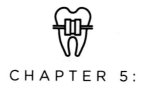

RETAINING THAT WINNING SMILE: RETAINERS, MAINTENANCE, AND THE DANGERS OF QUICK-FIX SOLUTIONS

Hello, Dear Reader! Chapter 5 *explores:*

- *Hold and Beautify: The Importance of Retainers*
- *Troubleshooting Orthodontic Problems: A Quickstep Guide*
- *What Are Those White Marks that Appear Sometimes after Braces Are Taken Off?*
- *Instant Braces? What about Veneers?*
- *Jessica's Story: Don't Let insurance Dictate Your Treatment*

As orthodontists, we consider straightening our patients' teeth as the most important step in treatment—but not the only one. We also need to collaborate with our patients in "maintaining" the results with retainers, which are either bonded (non-removable) or removable devices that can be taken out when eating and brushing.

We orthodontists have been searching since the profession started to find treatments that will help keep corrected teeth stay straight. It's our Holy Grail. Unfortunately, the best solutions we have at this point are retainers. The form of retainer will depend on what your doctor feels works best for your unique case. I try to let my patients have some input as to the type of retainer. For example, they might want a bonded retainer, because they don't feel they will be compliant with a removable retainer. If so, that's what I'll give them.

Whatever the case, retention isn't a one-size-fits-all proposition. Nothing works 100 percent for every person. That's why we don't just give you your retainers and say, "Take care. Have a nice life." We monitor the correction of your teeth over at least a year to ensure everything is staying in place and coming together correctly.

When everything looks good, then the responsibility for upkeep is turned over to *you*. Night wear of removable retainers will be needed for life. After a few years, wearing your retainer one or two nights a week is usually sufficient. If you stop wearing your retainer, then there is a chance that your teeth can slip out of alignment, as teeth tend to move as we age. The lower front teeth are the worst offenders.

Should you bristle at the thought of holding on to your retainer, think of it this way: If you lost twenty pounds and all you had to do to keep from regaining them was to put a magic lotion on before going to bed, you would do that, wouldn't you? Think of your retainer as your magic lotion.

HOLD AND BEAUTIFY: THE IMPORTANCE OF RETAINERS

I sometimes hear patients say, "The orthodontist took my braces off too soon and my teeth moved." The truth is that their braces weren't taken off too soon; they just weren't retained properly.

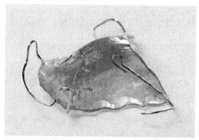

Fixed retainers are glued to your teeth and don't come out. Removable retainers can be taken out to eat and brush and floss. Fixed retainers are composed of a wire that is bonded (glued) to the back of your front teeth where it won't show. The most common type is attached to your lower front six

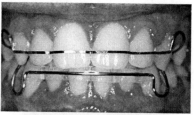

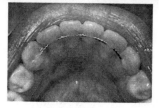

teeth, from canine to canine. Sometimes it's a solid, stiff wire and is only attached to the canines. Other doctors prefer a lighter, flexible wire that is attached to all the front teeth.

There are pros and cons to each retainer. The main advantage of a bonded retainer is that you don't have to remember to wear it. The down side is that it takes more effort to keep it clean. You need to use a flossing aid to floss between those teeth. The more teeth that are attached to the retainer wire, the harder they can be to clean. They can also come loose, if you bite into something that is particularly hard or sticky, like a candy apple.

In the old days, fixed retainers consisted of a heavy stainless steel wire soldered to bands that were cemented to the canines or the premolars directly behind the canines. These are very sturdy retainers and will stand up to just about anything. The problem is that you will have two noticeably silver teeth. Most orthodontists have transitioned to using bonded retainers, but I still run across people with banded retainers. These tend to be used by older orthodontists.

There are several types of removable retainers. The most common is called a Hawley retainer, which is made of acrylic plastic that covers the roof of your mouth and a wire that goes across your front teeth. This retainer has been around for more than one hundred years.

There are also usually some clasps that hold the retainer in. The retainer can be adjusted to move your teeth slightly. This type of retainer was often used in the past, because braces consisted of bands around each tooth, but when the braces were removed, there were spaces left. A retainer was needed that would allow these spaces to close. When orthodontists started bonding brackets to the teeth, we no longer had to deal with these spaces.

Today, a more popular type of retainer is called, simply enough, a "clear retainer." It's similar to an Invisalign tray and works by holding the teeth in place. In my practice, I recommend that clear retainers be worn full time for one month after braces are removed—and then should be worn only while sleeping. There are some advantages to the clear retainers. One is that they can be used as bleaching trays to bleach your teeth. Another is that they will protect your teeth if you tend to grind them while you sleep.

Both clear retainers and the Hawley retainers do a good job of keeping teeth straight. Some people just don't like the feeling of plastic covering their teeth; they prefer the Hawley retainer, which has plastic covering the roof of the mouth.

However, the Hawley retainer is more difficult to get used to and can cause some issues with clarity of speech. Some orthodontists—

particularly the ones using Hawley retainers—have their patients wear their retainer full time for a year. I personally prefer to go to night wear as soon as possible, as I've found that wearing a retainer full time increases the chances of something bad happening to it (tossed in the trash). Remember, in orthodontics, there are often many acceptable forms of treatment, so make sure you're satisfied with your treatment.

TROUBLESHOOTING ORTHODONTIC PROBLEMS: A QUICKSTEP GUIDE

Fortunately, there really aren't that many true orthodontic emergencies. The most common issues that arise with braces generally have to do with a loose bracket or band or a wire poke. If anything, they tend to be more of a nuisance than a true emergency, but they can, indeed, ruin a weekend. Here are some examples:

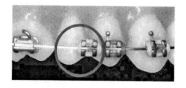

Loose Brackets and Bands: A loose bracket will usually just slide on the wire, becoming out of place. When this happens, my patients simply call and make an appointment for repairs. Should a band come loose, you should try to save it. It can be re-cemented at our office.

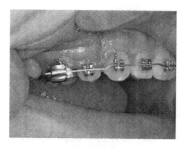

Pokes and Scrapes: If there is something poking or irritating your lips or cheeks, it should be covered up with orthodontic wax, which your orthodontist should give you. If not, you can find some at most drug stores. Because the wax is soft, you can form it into a ball—at least the size of a large pea—and "mold over" the irritation. Should the wax be too dense, you can soften it by kneading it or placing it in warm water.

Arch Wire Movements: Sometimes the arch wire of your braces can shift to one side or the other, which may cause it to poke your cheek. You can fix this yourself by shifting the wire back in place with some tweezers. Another option is to try clipping the end of the wire with some fingernail clippers.

Generally speaking, I define a true orthodontic emergency as any time a patient suffers trauma to the mouth and teeth. I've seen the results of catching a ball with your face, and it's not pretty. The good news is that in many cases, having braces can prevent a tooth from being completely knocked out of your mouth. If you have, however, had one of your teeth knocked out, it's imperative that you try to find it, so it can be placed back into your mouth and saved!

In collision trauma, the orthodontic wires of your braces can be bent and often need to corrected or replaced. You may need an X-ray to check for damage to the bone or roots. If you can't get hold of your dentist or orthodontist, you can go to the emergency room, particularly if there are cuts to the lips or cheeks.

WHAT ARE THOSE WHITE MARKS THAT SOMETIMES APPEAR AFTER BRACES ARE TAKEN OFF?

The white marks left on teeth after a person has his or her braces removed are called *demineralizations*. That occurs is when acid from bacteria in plaque starts to dissolve the enamel. It's the initial stage of the formation of a cavity, and it's totally preventable by good oral hygiene and by limiting the consumption of food with a lot of processed carbohydrates (sugar). The biggest offender is soda pop. We orthodontists try to prevent these white marks by making sure patients have the tools to properly clean their teeth. Our patients get a Sonicare toothbrush. We give them Prevident toothpaste, which has extra fluoride. We put a sealant on the surface of the teeth. At each appointment, if the teeth aren't clean, we go over how to clean them, over and over again if necessary. We do every-

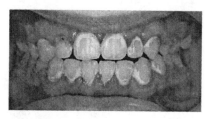

thing but go to your house, brush your teeth for you, and knock the can of Mountain Dew out of your hand. When I take someone's braces off and see white marks, it sends a dagger to my heart—but if you want to know who is to blame, you only have to look in the mirror.

The good news is that these demineralizations tend to fade after the braces are removed. If there are still noticeable white marks on your teeth a month after your braces are removed, tooth bleaching can make them much less noticeable, and you'll have whiter teeth. There are other treatments for white marks, all the way up to doing tooth-colored fillings or veneers to cover them up. But, of course, the best thing is to prevent them in the first place. Brush your teeth!

	pH	SUGAR AMOUNT
Water	7.00	0
Sprite	3.42	9.0
Diet Coke	3.39	0
Mountain Dew	3.22	11.0
Orange Slice	3.12	11.9
Diet Pepsi	3.05	0
Nestea	3.04	5.0
Gatorade	2.95	3.3
Coke	2.53	9.3
Pepsi	2.49	9.8
Battery Acid	1.00	0

INSTANT BRACES? WHAT ABOUT VENEERS?

Some dentists advocate having veneers placed over crooked front teeth as an alternative to orthodontic treatment, even though veneers cost as much or more than traditional orthodontic treatments and can yield some long-term challenges.

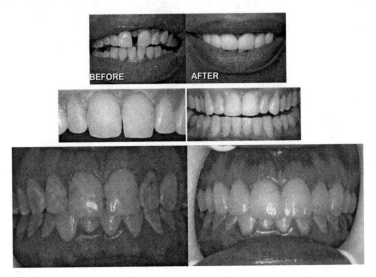

A veneer is like a false fingernail that is glued to the front of one or more of your teeth. The process involves reduction of the front of the teeth, an impression or digital scan, followed by the creation, in a lab, of porcelain veneers, which fit on the prepared teeth.

The advantage of getting veneers is that the work can be completed very quickly. Impressions are taken during your first visit. Then the veneers are cemented into place during the next. The time between visits depends on the speed of the lab. Because the position of the teeth is not changed, retainers are not needed.

Veneers can be a good idea if your teeth are malformed or discolored, which often occurs when certain antibiotics are given while your teeth are forming. Tetracycline is the most common cause of drug-related tooth discoloration. Fortunately, physicians are now aware of this problem and avoid giving tetracycline to young patients.

It's also true that some people just have unusual-looking teeth. Some are too small. They are overly tapered so that they are wider at the base of the tooth rather that the incisal edges, which gives the impression that they have spaces between their teeth even though they are touching each other near their gums.

In some cases, a patient's lateral incisors, which vary in shape and size more than any other teeth in your mouth, can present problems. If you have a "pegged lateral," for example, your tooth is very small and pointed. It is shaped like a teepee or an ice cream cone. This is a hereditary condition and is impossible to avoid in some families.

If your teeth are very crooked, your veneers may be quite thick. This makes it difficult to keep the gums healthy. In other cases, reductions become so significant that root canals may be required.

Veneers can also be fragile. They can chip or pop off, especially if your dentist had to remove most of the enamel from your tooth. If you have a deep bite or are a tooth grinder, you are more at risk for failure. Even under the best conditions you may need to have them remade periodically.

It's my opinion, therefore, that if your teeth are of acceptable shape and color, then orthodontic treatment is clearly the better option.

Jessica's Story: Don't Let Insurance Dictate Your Treatment

I first saw Jessica when she was a young girl and laid out a step-by-step plan for how to help straighten her teeth. But due to financial constraints, her mother decided to take her to an orthodontist who accepted her state insurance. The terms of the insurance paid for two years of orthodontic treatment, so after two years, her orthodontist said that her braces had done their job and were ready to come off. Jessica's mom was not quite sure and returned to me for an evaluation. The results were troubling. The orthodontist had removed four of Jessica's permanent teeth and was in the process of closing the spaces in her mouth, but had, at the same time, retracted her front teeth so far that they were actually tipped backwards. These procedures resulted in a "dished-in" profile (where the lips are sunken in, making the nose and chin prominent) with no lip support.

Unfortunately, this had made her look like a sixty-year-old woman with no teeth. In addition, one of the upper molars was moved so far forward that it was pushed up against her canine (eyetooth). The bicuspid that was supposed to sit between her molar and canine was left impacted in the roof of her mouth. Without making disparaging remarks about the treating orthodontist, I listed all the problems I saw remaining.

Before I finished, the mom was in tears. I ended up accepting Jessica into my practice and finishing her treatment at no cost to her parents. Her treatments ended up taking twice as long as needed, and she had teeth removed that didn't need to be removed. There's a lesson to be found here: If you have any question about the appropriateness of the recommended treatment, *get a second opinion!*

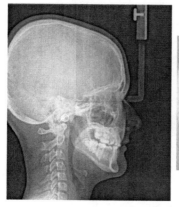 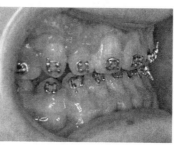

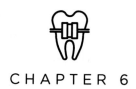

CHAPTER 6

AN EARLY START: THE IMPORTANCE OF ORTHODONTICS FOR YOUNG CHILDREN

Hello, Dear Reader! Chapter 6 explores:

- *What Is an Impacted Tooth?*
- *Crooked Teeth and the Bullying Effect*
- *Anna's Story: The Importance of Early Orthodontic Treatments*
- *Better Breathing, ADHD, and Eliminating Airway Obstructions*
- *Space Maintenance*
- *Breaking Bad Habits: The Dangers to Children Who Suck Their Thumbs*
- *What Is Palatal Expansion?*
- *A Primer on Headgear and Night Braces*
- *What Are Some Alternatives to Headgear?*

The American Association of Orthodontists has a snappy little slogan called "See You at Seven," which I hope all parents will keep in mind as their children begin making their way through elementary school.

The goal of the campaign is to encourage parents to have their children evaluated by an orthodontist at age seven, which is a particularly noteworthy year in the development of children's teeth.

It's around this time that children's six-year molars are in, and their incisors are either in or on their way in. Should serious problems begin to emerge, they can be identified at this point. The good news is that identifying issues early on allows us to launch interventions that will dramatically reduce the amount of discomfort, dental work, and treatments later on.

Should these problems be left to fester until a child enters his or her teen years, young patients could find themselves with impacted teeth, resorbed roots of permanent teeth, and conditions that could require removal of permanent teeth and even jaw surgery to correct.

Unfortunately, there are many dental professionals who are unaware that age seven is such a critical juncture in the development of a child's teeth. They incorrectly assume that they should wait until all of a child's baby teeth have come out before they send him or her to an orthodontist.

You don't need a referral from your dentist. You can be proactive and schedule an orthodontic appointment for your child yourself. It takes the burden off dentists, who are trained to look for dental decay and gum issues as opposed to monitoring growth and development.

In this way, subtle problems will be discovered early, and if treatment is needed, it can be done at the most opportune time, thus preventing (or alleviating) a whole host of issues, from ADHD symptoms and sleep disturbances to psychosocial problems like low self-esteem and bullying.

WHAT IS AN IMPACTED TOOTH?

Let's begin with a basic definition: An impacted tooth is one that has not properly erupted (emerged) into your arch. Most often you hear about impacted wisdom teeth, but often our upper canines (i.e. your "eyeteeth") can become impacted as well, as they are the last teeth to emerge.

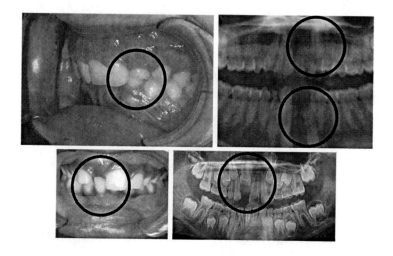

If, for example, you have severe crowding in your mouth, your eyeteeth are the ones that have the most difficulty finding space to come in. Their position in your jaw doesn't make things any easier. Because they start developing under your eyes (thus the name), they also have a lot farther to go and can run into several obstacles along the way.

When confronted with an impacted tooth, it's important for orthodontists to identify exactly where it is running into an obstruction. Upper canines can be mislocated in one's palate, the roof of one's mouth, or on the outer part of the jaw adjacent to your lips or cheeks. A panoramic X-ray allows us to determine if the tooth is impacted, but I can sometimes tell more about the impaction, such as whether it's on the tongue side or cheek side, by feeling around for a bulge in your gums. From there, the best way to determine exactly where the impacted tooth is located is to take a 3-D cone-beam scan.

There are a multitude of factors that can lead to an impacted tooth. Some are caused by crowding, others by baby teeth that don't fall out at the right time, and still others by benign tumors or hereditary factors.

Oftentimes, something as simple as expanding a patient's upper arch or removing his or her baby canines can prevent adult canines from becoming impacted. This is another reason for seeing the orthodontist sooner rather than later.

Often, when I see teens or adult patients with impacted upper canines, I can still see their baby canines sitting there, blocking the way. I always have to wonder why their dentists didn't remove them when they were younger. Everyone expects the baby teeth to fall out when they are ready. But if a permanent tooth isn't in the right place, the baby version may never come out on its own.

Inevitably it all comes down to this: The sooner an impacted tooth is identified, the better the chance that we can find a way to get it to erupt into the arch properly.

CROOKED TEETH AND THE BULLYING EFFECT

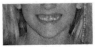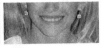 Unfortunately, I've seen more than my fair share of young patients who have been bullied and belittled because of crooked teeth and jagged smiles. Often parents will pull me aside and tell me how their children have been harassed, teased, and called all sorts of names, from "Bucky Beaver" to "SpongeBob SquarePants."

Simply put, there is no reason for your child to have to endure such cruelty. A short round of orthodontic treatments can often have him or her looking "normal" and boost his or her self-esteem to the point where the bullying will cease. On the other hand, if a child with "funny-looking teeth" isn't bothered by them, we can wait, monitor the situation, and correct it later.

Here are some common issues in children that lead to crooked teeth:

Crowding: Jumbled-up teeth and teeth erupting in strange places or without a place to go cause a great deal of concern but are easy to identify. As orthodontists, we want to make sure that a child's permanent teeth come in at the proper time and the right place. We can help by recommending the removal of baby teeth or by performing early treatments to help make room for new teeth. These procedures can prevent teeth from becoming impacted or causing damage to the roots of adjacent teeth.

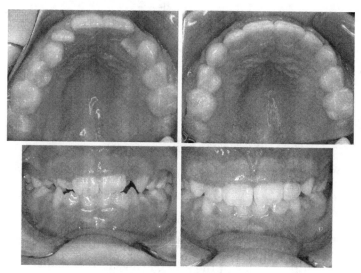

(L) Before. (R) After.

Severely Protrusive Teeth: A child with upper front teeth that stick out too far is not only at greater risk for ridicule but also has a greater propensity to seriously damage his or her teeth during a fall. Many times, a child's lower lip gets trapped behind the protrusive upper front teeth, which in turn keeps the front teeth sticking out and the lower teeth tipped backward. Often, these protrusions are accompanied by what we call a "deep bite," which is when an individual's lower front teeth are hitting the roof of his or her mouth and causing damage to the gums. Problems like this can usually be vastly improved with a year or less of treatment and intervention.

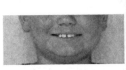
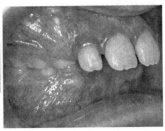

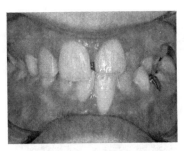

The anterior cross bite has caused recession of the gums. The posterior cross bite has caused the lower midline to shift to the patient's left.

Cross Bites: It's critical to correct cross bites as soon as they are discovered, particularly if they are causing a shift in one's bite. If a child has an anterior cross bite and must shift his or her lower jaw forward to bite down, this unnatural motion can stunt the growth of the upper jaw, in addition to wearing down the teeth and causing recession of the gums. If the cross bite involves the back teeth, there is often a shift to one side or the other. Either way, with an abnormal bite, one's jaw muscles must work overtime to chew, which can lead to TMJ problems. It can also, in children, affect the growth of their faces, making their lower jaws skew off to one side. Sometimes a cross bite is due to an underdeveloped upper jaw. If it is addressed early enough, the upper jaw can be moved forward, thus preventing the need for jaw surgery later.

Ankylosed Teeth: Simply put, ankylosis is a condition in which a tooth is fused to the bone. Unfortunately, ankylosed teeth cannot be moved orthodontically. They often need to be removed by the dentist or, in extreme cases, in conjunction with an oral surgeon. In addition, ankylosed teeth do not grow. This is not usually a problem in an adult mouth. In young people, however, both the teeth and jawbones grow upward from the lower jaw and downward from the upper jaw, which makes an ankylosed tooth appear to be sinking down into their gums. If the ankyloses occurs early in a child's life, the ankylosed tooth can be completely covered by gum tissue. Because ankylosed teeth don't usually fall out on their own, they can create a dip in one's dental arch and can cause incoming permanent teeth to become impacted or erupt out of position. Fortunately, with early identification, the ankylosed baby teeth can be removed at a time when it is not too difficult to remove and before it causes significant problems.

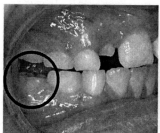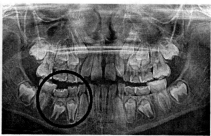

Ankylosed baby teeth.

ANNA'S STORY: THE IMPORTANCE OF EARLY ORTH-ODONTIC TREATMENTS

Anna is a beautiful little girl—with an impeccable fashion sense—who was eight years old when she first started treatments with me. Every time she walked into my office, she always wore wonderful, color-coordinated outfits, complete with matching accessories. The one thing that Anna *didn't* do willingly was smile. She was too embarrassed about the huge space between her front teeth. She told me, early in our visits, that her classmates called her SpongeBob, so she developed ways of not showing anyone her teeth. In essence, she found ways not to smile.

Fortunately, with six months of early treatment, we were able to provide her the winning smile that she longed so desperately to have—one that matched her impressive sense of style. Later, Anna and her mom told me that without question her treatments were worth every penny, as evidenced by the joy that radiated every time she curled her lips into her newfound perfect grin.

BETTER BREATHING, ADHD, AND ELIMINATING AIRWAY OBSTRUCTIONS

If your child is suffering from snoring or breathing difficulties, sometimes the issue can be aggravated by their teeth. In children, airway obstructions are usually caused by enlarged tonsils and adenoids, which can obstruct normal breathing through the nose. But sometimes these difficulties are made worse by a narrow jaw and lack of space for the tongue. Orthodontic treatment can easily widen the upper jaw, which in turn widens the floor of the nose, making it easier to breathe through one's nose and creates more room for the tongue.

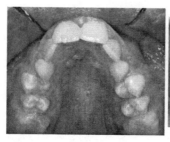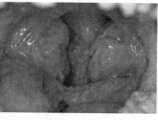

(L) Narrow upper jaw. (R) Enlarged tonsils.

Being able to breathe well, particularly while sleeping, is critical to a child's development, as sleep is a time when recent experiences are converted to long-term memories. Children who do not sleep well can exhibit a whole host of problems including struggles at school, stunts in growth, bedwetting, or possibly Attention Deficit/ Hyperactivity Disorder (ADHD).

Often, they don't need to be medicated; they just need a good night's rest. Children who sleep poorly can also suffer from a failure to thrive.

Parents should know that children should never snore, and children don't snore like adults; sometimes it sounds like a gentle "purr." If your child has problems breathing through his or her nose and has a narrow jaw, he or she should be evaluated first by a pediatrician or ENT doctor and then by an orthodontist, who may be able to help solve the issue.

Space Maintenance

If baby teeth are lost early, it may be a good idea to consider something we call a "space maintainer." One of the primary functions of baby teeth is to reserve space for the development of permanent teeth coming in behind them. If a baby tooth is lost before a permanent tooth is ready to come in, other teeth can drift into that space. This can cause an unerupted tooth to become impacted or to erupt in a strange position, including the roof of one's mouth or toward a cheek. Space maintainers hold the space open for adult teeth to emerge.

Proper space maintenance can prevent the need for removal of permanent teeth and make any future orthodontic treatments much simpler.

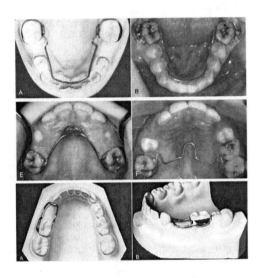

BREAKING BAD HABITS: THE DANGERS TO CHILDREN WHO SUCK THEIR THUMBS

Although often written off as a normal stage in a child's development, when a child sucks his or her thumb for a prolonged period, it can lead to a number of serious dental issues, including narrowed upper arches, cross bites, protrusive upper front teeth, and open bites.

Usually I tell my patients there's no reason to be concerned until children start to develop their permanent front teeth, around age five or six. If the habit persists, however, it can lead to problems that will require correction.

That being said, it is easier to quit smoking cigarettes than stop a thumb-sucking habit. Children (and adults for that matter) suck their thumb for the same reasons that people smoke: It's a stress-reliever. It releases endorphins, so when parents start scolding children for sucking their thumbs, their stress increases as does their desire to suck their fingers, creating a vicious circle.

For that reason, I often suggest that parents encourage positive behavior rather than punish bad behavior. Creating incentives certainly helps, such as providing your child with some easily attainable goals. For instance, if the child can refrain from thumb sucking for a few hours every afternoon for a week, then he or she earns a reward. The key, I've found, is to create manageable challenges that kids have a good chance of achieving.

Fortunately, a good orthodontist can help children who show a *willingness* to stop sucking their thumbs but lack the appropriate *willpower*. We have many different appliances that can be used not only to correct the narrowness of a patient's upper jaw but also help break the thumb-sucking habit.

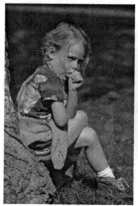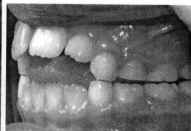

Anterior open bite and posterior cross bite that can result from a thumb or finger-sucking habit.

One appliance looks a bit like a car grill and physically prevents wearers from sticking their fingers or thumbs into their mouths. There are other options as well, but I caution you to be wary of removable appliances, which allow kids to remove them and start sucking their thumbs when no one is looking.

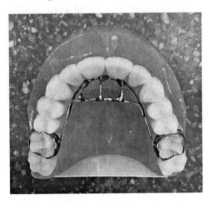

Habit appliance

Cemented appliances need to be in place for a year; it takes this long to make sure the habit doesn't come back.

It's important to know, however, that there is no appliance that can stop a child who doesn't want to stop. It will be an exercise in frustration.

I once saw a young woman who sucked her thumb up until the age of eighteen, which created an overbite so large you could practically drive a truck through it. Her mother took her to an orthodontist who put braces on her and used an appliance to help her stop sucking her thumb. However, she removed the braces and the appliance herself....

She finally stopped the habit of her own will when she got artificial nails (which she paid for) and didn't want to ruin them. The key is to find out what motivates a person.

WHAT IS A PALATAL EXPANSION?

Although the prospect of widening your child's upper jaw (what we call a palatal expansion) may sound, at first, like a pretty intrusive procedure, it's important to understand the anatomy involved.

The human upper jaw is composed of two halves, which are split down the middle by a suture. In young people, that suture is open, making it easy to manipulate the two halves. This is one of the reasons why, as Willy Wonka says, children are "so springy." As a child matures into an adult, that suture tends to close.

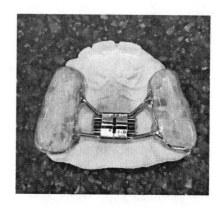

There are a variety of appliances we can use to separate the two halves of upper jaws in younger people all the way up into the teenage years and thus widen the bones of the upper jaw.

A rapid palatal expander (or rapid maxillary expander) is an adjustable appliance used to correct an upper jaw that is too narrow. It is cemented to the upper teeth, and parents are given the responsibility of adjusting it once or twice a day. Each quarter turn makes the appliance wider by .25 millimeters, thus separating the two halves of the upper jaw. As invasive as it might sound, these expanders are relatively painless. There will be a momentary feeling of pressure when it is turned, but the sensation goes away after just a few minutes.

One sign that the appliance is working is that a space will develop between the two front teeth, because these teeth are on either side of the suture. The expansion will continue until the upper jaw is slightly over-expanded. Then the expansion screw will be stabilized so it doesn't move. The expander is then left in place so that bone can fill in. During this stabilization phase, the gap between the patient's front teeth tends to close spontaneously, as the elastic fibers that connect our teeth pull our front teeth back together.

After approximately three months, the expander can be removed and a retainer made to be worn at night.

One thing to keep in mind: Even though expansion is often done at an early age, more expansion may be needed at the time when full braces are needed. In addition, these devices can also be used in adults, usually in conjunction with surgery that demands cuts to bones.

A PRIMER ON HEADGEAR AND NIGHT BRACES

I think most people are familiar with the dreaded headgear—that ungainly strap that kids have to put around their heads or necks when they sleep. For most, it's symbolic of nerds and the un-cool.

Headgear is primarily used to achieve an orthopedic effect on the upper jaw (maxilla) to correct children with an "overbite." As our faces grow, our jaws grow down and forward. If a child has a class II malocclusion (an overbite), then the forward growth of the upper jaw can be held back to allow the lower jaw's forward growth to catch up.

The headgear needs to be worn eight to twelve hours per day, mainly while sleeping.

Now to the big question: Does it work? Absolutely! But only if it's worn every night for the required amount of time, when a child is still growing, which is why the best time for headgear is right before puberty.

Unfortunately, girls and boys mature at different times. Often a girl goes through puberty before she is finished losing her baby teeth. And should a dentist wait for every one of a patient's baby teeth to be lost before a trip to the orthodontist, then our window of opportunity closes. If most growth has already occurred, then treatment options are limited to removing teeth or performing jaw surgery to correct the "overbite."

There are several different types of headgear. The type used depends on which direction the orthodontist wants to restrict the growth of the upper jaw. The most common type is called cervical-pull headgear, because the strap goes around the neck. Another type is the high-pull headgear where the strap fits on top of the head rather than the neck. The director of my orthodontic program, Dr. Charles Smith, used to lament about how, in the 1960s, the bouffant hairdo killed the high-pull headgear. Today, we don't run across too many bouffants—though headgear itself is just about as endangered. There is nothing wrong with an orthodontist wanting to treat your child with a headgear, but be aware that there are alternatives.

WHAT ARE SOME ALTERNATIVES TO HEADGEAR?

Let's be honest. Today's young people are very busy, and having the time and inclination to wear a headgear for the required amount of time can be difficult. We orthodontists have a joke, "I use headgear, but my patients don't". Should headgear prove to be too cumbersome, there are a few alternatives that are worth discussing:

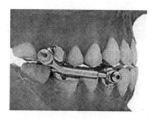

The Herbst Appliance: Named after a German orthodontist from the 1930s, this appliance is attached to one's teeth and placed entirely inside the mouth. It consists of telescoping rods that position the lower jaw forward when biting down. Initially it was thought that this appliance increased the growth of the lower jaw, but it actually works by holding back the forward growth of one's upper jaw, just like headgear. Its principal advantage is that orthodontists never have to wonder how well the patient is wearing the appliance. It's glued in, so there is nothing to put in or take out.

Removable Functional Appliances: These devices go by several names, including the Activator, the Bionator, The Frankel appliance, and the Twin Block. These appliances are made of plastic and wire, similar to a retainer. They're usually removed when eating, and worn for different lengths of time depending on the case and device. They work similarly to the Herbst appliance in that they force the person to bite in a forward position. They must be worn in order to work, though, and so are heavily dependent on the cooperation of the patient.

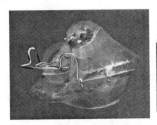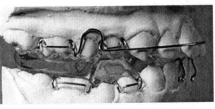

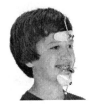**Reverse-Pull Facemask:** This is one form of headgear that is still quite popular among orthodontists. A facemask is used to correct the opposite problem of an overbite—an underdeveloped upper jaw. In a child with an "underbite," it is used to pull the upper jaw out and sometimes in a downward direction. With a reverse-pull facemask, the sooner a patient starts, the better off he or she generally is. Children as young as five or six can benefit from this type of treatment and can possibly avoid jaw surgery in the future, should they wear it on a regular basis. There are some orthodontists who tell their patients to wear the facemask full-time for

three months. I just can't bring myself to ask my patients to wear a facemask to school, but if any kids would be willing to do that, more power to them; they would get corrected much quicker. It's easier to get a six- or seven-year-old to wear something like a facemask than get a twelve- or thirteen-year-old to wear a headgear.

In the end, it's important to remember one thing most of all: There are many orthodontic problems that should be identified and treated in children while the baby teeth are still present, and orthodontists are best qualified to perform these procedures. So, to be proactive and get the best care for your children, just remember those four golden words: "See you at seven."

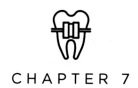

CHAPTER 7

THE HIDDEN HEALTH BENEFITS OF ORTHODONTICS, AND OTHER ISSUES

Hello, Dear Reader! Chapter 7 explores:

- *Your Bite and Its Importance to Oral Health*
- *To Implant or Not to Implant*
- *Building a Better Bridge*
- *Mimi's Story: Always Discuss All Your Options*
- *Sleep Tight: A Novel Approach to Sleep Apnea*
- *Help, I've Got TMJ!*
- *Understanding Orthognathic Surgery*
- *Slenderizing Teeth: IPR, ARS, Enamelplasty*
- *Risks of Orthodontic Treatment*
- *What If We Have to Move?*

When properly administered, professional orthodontic treatments can produce far more than just aesthetic benefits. Although less often discussed, they can also generate a host of health benefits that cutting-edge research is just beginning to uncover.

While it's true that orthodontic treatments are often initiated to create a more beautiful smile, making your teeth properly fit together, we are ensuring that your jaw, teeth, and gums are functioning optimally as one complete unit. Thus, patients are often less susceptible to adverse tooth wear, the gums are at reduced risk of problems, and the temporomandibular (TMJ) joints avoid unwanted stress.

Surprisingly enough, many adults are still under the misconception that orthodontic treatment is only useful for children and teens. Nothing could be further from the truth, as proper orthodontic care can benefit patients of all ages, including adults who suffer from sleep issues, eating problems, and jaw pain.

THE IMPORTANCE OF GUM HEALTH

To put it simply, having straight teeth will greatly aid you in maintaining proper oral hygiene. Teeth that are well aligned are undoubtedly easier to brush and floss than severely crowded teeth. If you are missing a tooth, your adjacent teeth can lean into that space and try to fill it, creating issues involving supporting bones and gums.

In addition, untreated cross bites, deep bites, or open bites can have significant impacts on your dental health.

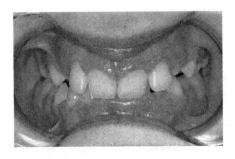

Deep Bite: A deep bite occurs when a patient has too much overlap of his or her front teeth. A deep bite can contribute to severe dental wear, to the point where the patient will need extensive restorative work, including crowns and even root canals.

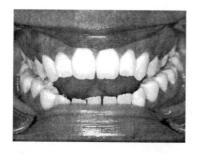

Open Bite: An open bite is the opposite of a deep bite. This emerges when a patient has no overlap of the front teeth when biting down. In severe cases, only the molars touch when biting, which makes it impossible to bite down into a sandwich or a slice of pizza. Patients who have an open bite often must use a fork and knife to cut everything they eat, not to mention a reduced ability to properly chew their food. Over the years, I've found that correcting an open bite often yields vast improvements in a patient's ability to enjoy daily life.

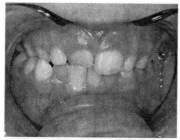
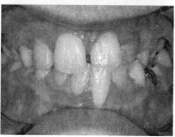

Cross Bite: As stated earlier, the upper teeth are supposed to overlap the lower teeth. If there is a lot of crowding or an incongruity in the width of your upper and lower jaws, then you could have what we call a cross bite, with some or all of the upper teeth trapped behind the lower teeth. Cross bites can cause a functional shift of your jaw to accommodate the fit of your teeth. Our jaw muscles learn how to open and shut the lower jaw for our teeth to physically fit together.

If your dentist can "wiggle" your lower jaw back to where your jaw joints are seated, and your bite is different from where you normally bite, then you have a shift. In some cases, your jaw muscles will not even allow your jaw to seat (i.e., bite down) properly and because they have been programmed to chew incorrectly for so long, they fight to close in a certain pattern so that the teeth won't be damaged.

The reason for this is that teeth have very sensitive proprioception (a tooth's way of signaling the brain that something is awry). They can detect very minute differences. A good example of this is how something as thin as a human hair is immediately detectable. Or, when you have some dental work done, any change seems enormous.

Putting a plastic splint (mouthguard) between a patient's teeth reduces the feeling of proprioception. All the little hills and valleys on the surface of the teeth are smoothed out so there is no best way to bite so that the teeth fit well. This allows your muscles to relax and lets your jaw fully seat. In this way, we can tell where a person's true bite is. We usually only do this for people with TMJ pain, but there are orthodontists who put all their adult patients in splints prior to performing orthodontic treatments to ensure that the jaws are properly seated.

Telescoping Cross Bite: In a normal bite, the cusps of the lower back teeth fit in the valley that's made by the cusps of the upper teeth. A telescoping cross bite occurs when the lower teeth miss the valley. If the teeth don't touch other teeth, then they simply continue to grow past each other. Correction is difficult, because the teeth need to be pushed up prior to correcting the cross bite. If the cross bite involves all or most of your teeth on one side, there is nothing to work with to make the correction. Sometimes a temporary anchorage device (TAD) is used. This is a tiny metal screw that is placed in the bone, which can then be used to move the teeth. In some cases, jaw surgery is required, which is another reason that early detection is important. It's easy for this to be missed by your dentist or hygienist. It's much easier to correct this type of problem when it's found early.

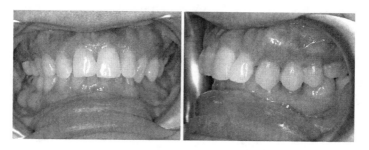

Telescoping crossbite on the left with resulting over eruption of the upper teeth.

TO IMPLANT OR NOT TO IMPLANT

Patients who are missing permanent teeth have an important decision to make concerning how they want to fill the gap in their mouths. There are several choices available to them.

Sometimes, a baby tooth is left remaining that can be preserved and maintained for long-term use. This usually occurs in the posterior of one's mouth, especially if a patient still has his or her primary molar in place of a missing second bicuspid. Such an arrangement can last a lifetime.

With missing front teeth, however, maintaining a patient's baby tooth is usually not an option. The baby incisor teeth are much smaller than the permanent teeth that replace them, so their roots are not very substantial. In addition, baby teeth with missing permanent successors are often lost when other permanent teeth erupt.

Often, these issues emerge with upper lateral incisors, the smaller teeth right next to the two front teeth in the middle of your mouth. There are two ways to deal with missing upper incisors: You either make room for some type of replacement or you close the space and substitute other teeth for those that are missing.

Closing this space usually involves moving a canine or "eyetooth" next to the central incisor and reshaping it to make it look it's a lateral incisor. How well this works, however, is wholly dependent on the shape of your canines. Sometimes a patient's canine is on the small side and lends itself to being reshaped, but if a canine is too large, then it may not look as aesthetically pleasing.

Over the years, I've found that substituting canines for missing lateral incisors is the best option, particularly if both of them are missing. There are some dentists who feel it's important to maintain the canine in the canine position for long-term health, thus they prefer that the space for the missing tooth or teeth be opened.

And yet sometimes it's just not practical to close a space, as the space needs to be opened for a replacement tooth. If this is the case, a decision must be made as to how the space will be filled.

In the United States, we tend to lean toward using implants. In this case, a metal cylinder is placed in your jawbone, to which a prosthetic tooth is attached. These implants are as close to natural teeth as you can get.

If you live in Europe, the transplantation of a tooth may be recommended. Bicuspids and even wisdom teeth have been successfully transplanted and reshaped to look like anterior teeth. The difference between an implant and a transplant is that an implant cannot be moved once it's in place. A transplanted tooth, however, can be moved orthodontically, just like any other regular tooth.

There is one other important thing to consider in terms of younger patients: In general, our teeth and jaws grow downward, so if an implant is placed in a patient who is still growing, it will look like the implant is sinking into his or her gums.

What is really happening, however, is that the natural teeth are growing downward, leaving the implant at the level in which it was originally placed. Implants can suffer from surrounding gum disease, just like natural teeth. And in some cases, the gray metal cylinders can show through the gum tissue and look unattractive. They can also fail or become damaged and have to be removed, which is often accompanied by the destruction of the supporting bone. This can eventually lead to bone grafting and gum surgery.

Why then, you may be asking, are implants generally used instead of transplants?

First and foremost, it's not always easy to find suitable teeth from donors for transplants. Ideally, this is a tooth where the root is a half to three-quarters formed. Transplants also require a proper root and a crown that can be recontoured, not to mention the fact that many surgeons in the United States are unfamiliar with performing such procedures.

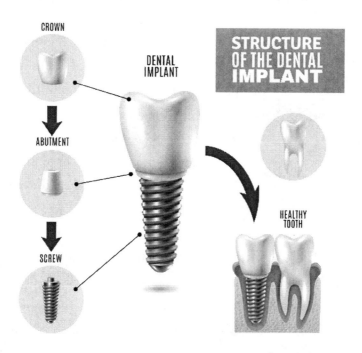

CROWN

DENTAL IMPLANT

STRUCTURE OF THE DENTAL IMPLANT

ABUTMENT

HEALTHY TOOTH

SCREW

BUILDING A BETTER BRIDGE

For those uninterested in either implants or transplants, there are other options to consider. Here is a short list:

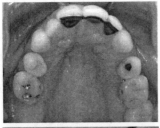

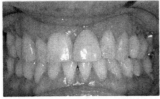

Maryland Bridge: A Maryland bridge is a false tooth that is attached to an existing tooth with "wings" that are glued to the backs of the teeth on each side of the missing tooth. These bridges, which cannot be removed by the patient, require minimal preparation and can be performed on teeth that are still growing. They are good options for teens who are planning on having dental implants in the future.

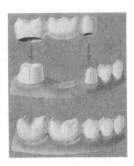

The teeth on the ends are prepared for crowns.

Conventional Bridge: A conventional bridge can be also applied. However, this procedure requires the teeth on either side of the missing tooth to be prepared for a crown, which involves considerable removal of tooth structure. If nearby teeth have significant fillings or are discolored, then conventional bridges are often the best choice.

Removable Appliance: This retainer-like appliance (often called a *flipper)* works in conjunction with an acrylic in the roof of one's mouth with a plastic tooth is attached to it. The downside, of course, is that these appliances are removable, which makes them prone to breaking and getting lost. Removable appliances are the most affordable way to replace a missing tooth, but they are usually considered a temporary solution.

One of the problems with opening a space for an implant in a growing patient is that it can be difficult to keep their teeth in the proper position for the placement of the implant. Surgeons need a certain amount of space between the roots of adjacent teeth to place an implant and should there be a considerable amount of time between when an orthodontic treatment is complete and an implant is placed, then the roots can move and get in the way.

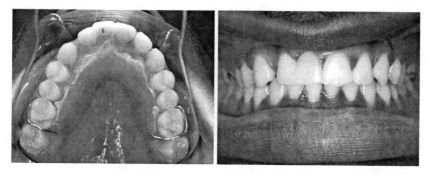

Flipper replacing the upper right front tooth.

Typical Hawley-type retainers are often insufficient to maintain the proper root position, and many times braces must be reapplied to correct the root position prior to implantation. As you can imagine, this can lead to very unhappy parents and patients.

In the end, it's safe to say that there are simply no substitutes for a natural tooth. Therefore, in my practice, I tend to close the space for missing teeth whenever possible rather than open up spaces for artificial replacements. There are more and more studies that show that this is the superior choice.

Linda's Story: Always Discuss All Your Options

I once saw an adult patient, Linda, who was missing her upper lateral incisors. She had bridgework on the upper front six teeth to replace the missing teeth. She also had an "overbite." We treated her by removing her fake teeth and bringing the protruding front teeth back, closing the space for the missing teeth. She will have new crowns made for her front teeth, and she will have a great smile—no "overbite" and no bridgework to deal with. I'm not sure if the dentist who did the bridgework initially discussed the possibility of orthodontic treatment to close the space, but there's a good chance it never crossed his mind.

SLEEP TIGHT: A NOVEL ORTHODONTIC APPROACH TO SLEEP APNEA

Being able to breathe well, particularly when sleeping, is a problem that is just beginning to gain the attention it deserves. Almost everyone knows someone with obstructive sleep apnea who uses a CPAP machine when sleeping. And if they don't, they probably know someone who snores like a lumberjack, which is a nuisance that not only irritates others but can also pose serious health risks.

Obstructive sleep apnea occurs when a person stops breathing during sleep. It often leads to daytime drowsiness as well as health problems, including high blood pressure, diabetes, heart disease, obesity, headaches, tooth grinding, and stroke.

Often sleep apnea occurs when your tongue falls to the back of your throat while you're sleeping, thus blocking off your airway. The body's desperate efforts to suck up air cause a flight-or-fight response, which leads to an increased heart rate and blood pressure. Often, the person awakes gasping for air, which is part of the reason why so many heart attacks occur early in the morning.

A good orthodontist can help make sure that your tongue has enough room in your mouth by widening your arches. In such cases, we tend not to have to do as many tooth extractions as we did in the past, as we've realized that removing teeth can narrow our patients' arches instead of widening them.

Today we can help alleviate many of the negative effects of snoring and sleep apnea in ways that were virtually unheard of years ago.

HELP, I'VE GOT TMJ!

It's important to note, right from the start, that *everyone* has TMJ, which stands for temporomandibular joint—a.k.a., the jaw joint. The proper term for problems associated with TMJ is temporomandibular dysfunction, or TMD.

There are a range of signs and symptoms that comprise TMD, including jaw pain, headaches, and a painful popping and clicking of the joint. In some patients, these problems come and go, and for others, they become chronic issues.

Often, stress is a principal motivating factor in the manifestation of TMD. People tend to clench their teeth together when they are stressed, which strains the face muscles and can damage the joint. In other cases, some form of trauma to one's jaw or head can contribute to TMD problems, including long dental procedures during which the jaw is kept open for extended periods of time, as well as issues stemming from the general anesthesia, car accidents, and sports injuries.

Sometimes, pain can emerge months or years after an injury occurs, but other instigating factors can lead to flare-ups of TMD.

Although there is still a great deal to learn about TMD, we have made some important discoveries. It was once thought, for example, that a "bad bite" was the primary cause of TMD. As a result, many people had their teeth reshaped or had crowns put in to treat TMD.

But now it is generally believed that a person's bite, while not completely unrelated to TMD, is not the primary cause of the condition.

Fortunately, there are many ways to treat TMD. There is no real consensus as to which procedures are most effective, but, in my opinion, non-invasive treatment should always be conducted before more invasive steps are taken.

Often the use of non-steroidal anti-inflammatory drugs (such as ibuprofen), the application of moist heat to the affected areas, and a soft diet can lead to successful outcomes. In addition, being aware of destructive habits such as clenching your teeth can be very helpful. Many people are not aware that most of the time our teeth should not be touching. Subsequent steps often involve some type of orthotic or night guard, which patients wear while they are sleeping.

More chronic forms of TMD require more aggressive treatment. In our office, we treat these patients using techniques derived from sports medicine. Your TMJ is a joint that can be injured in a similar way to an athlete's knee, which is why a comprehensive approach that relies on ultrasound, muscle manipulation, cold lasers, orthotics, and home care can be very successful.

UNDERSTANDING ORTHOGNATHIC SURGERY

Orthognathic surgery is performed to correct the skeletal relationships of one's jaws. Sometimes your upper or lower jaws are positioned too far forward; other times they're positioned too far backward. In addition, there can be issues stemming from too much of an overlap of a patient's front teeth, or no overlap at all. Often, we can correct these bites with braces alone, even when there are underlying skeletal problems.

In severe cases, however, the best approach usually involves a combination of braces and jaw surgery, with surgery performed by an oral and maxillofacial (jaw and face) surgeon.

Orthognathic surgery is often performed in cases where there is a severe deficiency of the lower jaw, which causes a person to look like he or she has a very small chin. In other cases, it's performed for patients whose lower jaw has grown too much, like the comedian Jay Leno. When these patients bite down, they have an underbite.

Orthodontists can often produce a satisfactory bite in a person with a small lower jaw, which can then be augmented by additional surgery performed for aesthetic reasons, if desired. Those with large lower jaws, however, often require surgery simply to get their bottom teeth into an acceptable relationship with their upper teeth.

There are orthodontists who do not want to do what they consider "compromise" treatments. If they feel that the best aesthetic results require surgery, they will only treat in conjunction with an oral surgeon. Personally, I believe in informing patients that there is a surgical option but not forcing the decision on them.

I don't want to insist on jaw surgery because of the significant risks involved with such procedures, including numbness of the lower lip and chin, infection, and even in rare cases, death (a risk of general anesthesia).

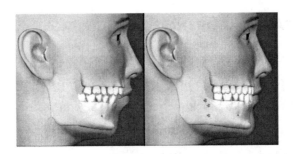

Example of jaw surgery to correct an "overbite."

SLENDERIZING TEETH: IPR, ARS, ENAMELPLASTY

Tooth *slenderizing* is a way of avoiding the removal of a tooth. The process entails gently removing a little bit of tooth enamel from several teeth. This is usually accomplished with a "drill," which has a bad reputation but can usually be used quite painlessly, even without anesthesia. These procedures go by many names, but the correct technical terms are interproximal reduction (IPR) and air-rotor stripping (ARS). Should these terms be too hard to recall, just remember the term "slenderizing," and your orthodontist will know what you mean.

The outer part of the crown of a tooth is made up of enamel, which is not only the hardest substance in the body but also contains no blood vessels or nerves. The thickness of the enamel on teeth varies from person to person, but we generally have 1.5 millimeters of enamel to work with. We can safely remove up to .5 millimeters of enamel from your teeth. However, the most that is typically removed is 0.25mm.

This procedure does not affect the health of your teeth, nor does it increase the likelihood of cavities. However, If your teeth are small to begin with, it will not help to have even skinnier teeth.

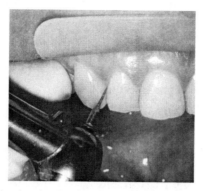

Interproximal reduction being done with a handpiece.

RISKS OF ORTHODONTIC TREATMENTS

The most common problems associated with orthodontic treatment are the white marks that can appear once braces are taken off. Fortunately, these white marks can often be prevented with good oral hygiene (just brush your teeth).

However, the problem that most concerns orthodontists is a phenomenon called *root resorption*, i.e. the shortening of the roots. A small amount of root resorption is to be expected and is insignificant. There is, however, a small percentage of people who experience a significant amount of root resorption, at which time half or more of the root disappears.

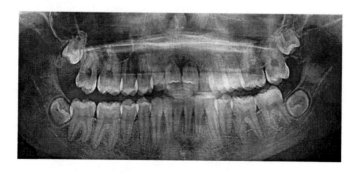

Root resorption of the upper front teeth.

We refer to this as *idiopathic* resorption, meaning we don't know why it happens. Sometimes root resorption can be caused by orthodontic treatments, such as using too much force or moving the roots into the crowns of unerupted teeth.

Those who are concerned about root reabsorption should choose Invisalign, which rarely leads to resorption, as the tooth movement is more controlled than with traditional braces.

Another problem we are always on the lookout for is old-fashioned periodontal, or "gum," problems. In the case of gum recession, the root of a tooth becomes exposed. This requires a visit to the periodontist, a gum specialist. Often, it can be corrected with a gum graft.

The far more common type of gum problem is simply an excess amount of gum tissue. Our gums can react to braces and less-than-perfect brushing by becoming swollen. This is particularly common in teenagers who are experiencing hormonal changes at the same time they are getting their teeth straightened.

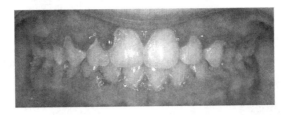

Swollen gums from poor oral hygiene.

The good news is that when their braces are removed, swelling usually goes away by itself. If it doesn't, it can be corrected with a soft-tissue laser, which many orthodontists today have in their offices.

WHAT IF WE HAVE TO MOVE?

We are a very mobile society, and people often have to move in the middle of an orthodontic treatment, sometimes to the next county or in other cases to a different country. Fortunately, your orthodontist has access to a directory of all the other orthodontists in the world. Therefore, if you give us a little notice, arrangements can be made for your treatments to be continued by an orthodontist in your new location.

During these transitions, there are various important things to consider. How much of the orthodontic treatment fee has been earned by the starting orthodontist? How much treatment is left, and how much will the continuing orthodontist charge? Orthodontic treatment is so varied, and there are so many different types of appliances and bracket systems, that it is highly unlikely that a new orthodontist will approach things in the exact same way as your initial orthodontist.

In general, orthodontists don't like treating transfer patients. Some just outright refuse to take them. Others insist on removing whatever braces the patient came in with and placing their own braces. This adds cost to the patient. As an orthodontist in the US Air Force, my primary job was treating patients who were relocated in the middle of their treatments. I had to treat a revolving door of transfer patients with whatever appliances they walked in with. Today, I still always try to work with whatever appliances my transfer patients come to me with. It's good for the patient, and it's good for our profession.

There are other issues that are going to make transfers more complicated. The first is Invisalign. As I mentioned earlier, there is a great disparity in the skill level and knowledge regarding Invisalign. There may not be a qualified Invisalign provider within two hundred miles of your new home. If you have an open-minded orthodontist, he or she should continue the existing Invisalign treatment your previous orthodontist started. However, the new person may insist on placing conventional braces. Placing braces on an Invisalign patient is going to cost the patient more.

An alternative is to continue seeing your original orthodontist from your new location. With Invisalign, if you are changing your aligners on schedule and are compliant, then you can see your orthodontist every few months instead of every six weeks. This may be an option, particularly if you have family in your original location and will be making visits there periodically.

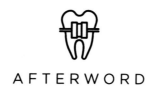

WHAT YOUR SMILE MEANS TO ME

I'd like to close by saying, as simply and as clearly as possible, that I am extremely thankful to be a member of this great profession, which positively impacts so many lives in so many ways.

I've seen how my work and the work of other orthodontists has helped countless people reclaim not only their smiles, but their confidence, self-esteem, and general health as well.

I truly believe that orthodontic treatment is one of the best values in health care, and I hope that, in some small way, the information and stories in this book will help you come to that same conclusion.

In choosing the right orthodontist—someone who is knowledgeable and will progress through the available options thoughtfully and strategically, all while listening to all your concerns—you will see the true value of healthy teeth and a healthy smile.

I would like to end on a personal note and tell you how I found my way into a profession I truly love and respect—not to mention how I found my way back to the community I call home.

As a young man, like many of my peers, I longed to get away and live where there was more action. I wanted to see the world. I went to school at the University of Maryland at College Park (Go Terps!). I then attended dental school at the University of Maryland Dental School in Baltimore, the first dental school in the world. After graduating *magna cum laude* from dental school, I joined the United States Air Force, where I did a one-year general practice residency, which is like an additional intense year of dental school.

We received in-depth training in oral surgery, root canals, doing crowns and fillings, and treating gum disease. I enjoyed my training, but the one thing we didn't learn was orthodontics.

Orthodontics is so different from all other aspects of dentistry that most dental schools only cover the bare minimum. That's why it became the first dental specialty. At the time, I thought that was fine. After all, I was a "real dentist." After my general-practice residency, I decided that I wanted to specialize in oral surgery.

Upon graduation, the Air Force sent me to RAF (Royal Air Force) Bentwaters in Great Britain to practice general dentistry. Because I was planning on applying for oral surgery, I did as much surgery as I could. Then, one day we had an oral pathologist visit and give us a day of continuing education.

We all went to lunch, and the topic of conversation turned to the various dental specialties. Somewhere along the line, the topic of orthodontics came up. "Oh, the orthodontists have it made!" the oral pathologist said. Orthodontics was one of those rare medical fields where people didn't mind coming to see you. Orthodontists didn't have to give people needles; they improved people's appearance; they worked with young people. At that very moment, it was like God spoke to me, "You shall become an orthodontist!"

I applied for and was accepted into Air Force-sponsored orthodontic training, which I completed at Emory University. It was two years of the most professionally gratifying education I ever experienced. I love dentistry, but I truly fell head-over-heels in love with orthodontics.

I love that there is no one right way to treat a patient. You can use different appliances, remove teeth or not remove teeth, and work in conjunction with oral surgeons to perform orthodontic and surgical treatment. Your principal aim is simply to satisfy your patients' needs.

It's also a profession that allows me to constantly expand my knowledge and skills, to continue to provide the best for my patients. It's one of the reasons I went through all the trouble and effort to become board certified. It's also why I'm proud to say I am among the top 1 percent of Invisalign providers in the United States. All these efforts translate into the highest quality of care for my patients.

It also provides my patients a greater array of treatment options, and it means I'm open to asking questions: Do you, for instance, want to be treated with Invisalign or traditional braces? I listen, and then collectively, we determine which option is best for you.

Old-fashioned as it may sound, I fundamentally believe that the more patience and attention I show my patients, the more my business will grow. If I give you a quality orthodontic experience, you are more likely to spread the word about my practice to friends and family.

That's one of the reasons I wrote this book. To educate and enlighten. To show people that it's going to be OK. That these treatments can, indeed, make a difference.

In the end, what I desire is simple. After sitting in my chair, I want my patients to go home and turn to their loved ones and say, "Oh, you've got to go to Dr. Crouse if you need braces."

Those are the kind of endorsements I believe in—and strive to earn every single day.

I hope *A Smile to Change Your Life* will direct you toward high-quality orthodontics work that that will last a lifetime. And for the parents reading this book: I want you to feel that you've made a great investment in your children's lives—one that will give them confidence and self-esteem and help them be successful in the world, not only today but in the years and decades to follow.

CPSIA information can be obtained
at www.ICGtesting.com
Printed in the USA
FFOW02n2045310118
44814448-44949FF